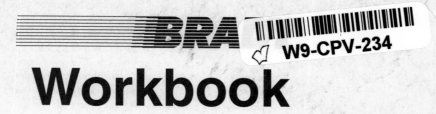

Workbook

J. DAVID BERGERON
CHRIS LE BAUDOUR

First Responder

8TH EDITION

J. DAVID BERGERON
CHRIS LE BAUDOUR

MEDICAL REVIEWER

KEITH WESLEY, MD

LEGACY AUTHOR

GLORIA BIZJAK

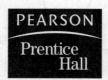

PEARSON

Prentice Hall

Upper Saddle River, New Jersey 07458

Publisher: Julie Levin Alexander
Publisher's Assistant: Regina Bruno
Executive Editor: Marlene McHugh Pratt
Acquisitions Editor: Sladjana Repic
Associate Editor: Monica Moosang
Senior Managing Editor for Development: Lois
    Berlowitz
Development Editor: Patricia Gillivan, Triple SSS Press
    Media Development
Director of Marketing: Karen Allman
Executive Marketing Manager: Katrin Beacom
Marketing Specialist: Michael Sirinides
Managing Editor: Patrick Walsh
Production Liaison: Julie Li
Production Editor: Peggy Hood
Manufacturing Manager: Ilene Sanford
Manufacturing Buyer: Pat Brown
Senior Design Coordinator: Christopher Weigand
Cover Photo: Ray Kemp/911 Imaging
Composition: Aptara
Printing and Binding: Bind-Rite Graphics
Cover Printer: Phoenix Color Corporation

Notice on Care Procedures

It is the intent of the authors and publisher that this manual be used as part of a formal Emergency Medical Responder education program taught by qualified instructors and supervised by a licensed physician. The procedures described in this manual are based upon consultation with appropriate medical authorities. The authors and publisher have taken care to make certain that these procedures reflect currently accepted clinical practice; however, they cannot be considered absolute recommendations.

The material in this manual contains the most current information available at the time of publication. However, federal, state, and local guidelines concerning clinical practices, including, without limitation, those governing infection control and universal precautions, change rapidly. The reader should note, therefore, that new regulations may require changes in some procedures.

It is the responsibility of the reader to familiarize himself or herself with the policies and procedures set by federal, state, and local agencies as well as the institution or agency where the reader is employed. The authors and the publisher of this textbook and the supplements written to accompany it disclaim any liability, loss, or risk resulting directly or indirectly from the suggested procedures and theory, from any undetected errors, or from the reader's responsibility to stay informed of any new changes or recommendations made by any federal, state, and local agency as well as by his or her employing institution or agency.

Notice on Gender Usage

The English language has historically given preference to the male gender. Among many words, the pronouns, "he" and "his" are commonly used to describe both genders. Society evolves faster than language, and the male pronouns still predominate our speech. The authors have made great effort to treat the two genders equally, recognizing that a significant percentage of Emergency Medical Responders are female. However, in some instances, male pronouns may be used to describe both males and females solely for the purpose of brevity. This is not intended to offend any readers.

Pearson Prentice Hall™ is a trademark of Pearson Education, Inc.
Pearson® is a registered trademark of Pearson plc.
Prentice Hall® is a registered trademark of Pearson Education, Inc.
Pearson Education, Ltd., *London*
Pearson Education Australia Pty. Limited, *Sydney*
Pearson Education Singapore Pte. Ltd.
Pearson Education North Asia Ltd., *Hong Kong*
Pearson Education Canada, Ltd., *Toronto*

Pearson Educación de Mexico, S.A. de C.V.
Pearson Education—Japan, *Tokyo*
Pearson Education Malaysia, Pte. Ltd.
Pearson Education, Upper Saddle River, New Jersey

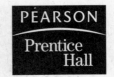

10 9 8 7 6 5 4 3
ISBN-10:   0-13-244747-9
ISBN-13: 978-0-13-244747-8

CONTENTS

Appendices

PREFACE

This workbook is meant to accompany the First Responder, 8th edition, textbook. Many of its features allow you to work at your own pace, helping you to evaluate your progress through a formal Emergency Medical Responder course. As you become aware of a weakness, this workbook will help you to correct that problem. Should you still have difficulty with certain materials, you will be able to go to your instructor and state specifically what your problem is and what kind of help you need.

To benefit from this workbook, you will have to follow the procedures stated here. Your instructor may direct you to skip certain exercises or assign additional exercises. It is hoped that you will put your time and efforts into each chapter as directed. Not only will you benefit, but so will those to whom you provide Emergency Medical Responder-level emergency care.

No attempt has been made to cover all the material presented in the textbook. You will find that this workbook has been designed to review the most significant areas of emergency care and to highlight those areas that may be overlooked during your first reading of the textbook. The workbook is not meant to replace your instructor's classes, the textbook, or the skills laboratories. In other words, this workbook is not meant to be a substitute for a well-designed Emergency Medical Responder course.

Each chapter of this workbook requires you to complete eight steps. Leaving out one of these steps or hurrying through any one of them will significantly reduce your learning. The eight steps you must follow are:

Step 1. There are two parts to Step 1. Each chapter has a Reading Assignment from the textbook. This assignment includes a list of objectives. Before beginning the assigned reading, go through the entire list of objectives. These objectives will tell you the things you should know and be able to do before completing each unit of study. Once you have read the objectives, complete the reading assignment. As you read through the chapter, keep a list of those terms you do not understand or feel will be difficult for you to remember. Do *not* attempt to do any of the exercises until you have read the entire assignment given here or assigned by your instructor.

Step 2. After you have completed the reading assignment, reread the objectives, making certain that you can relate what you have read in the chapter to specific objectives.

Step 3. The third step is the Key Terms & Definitions section. Using your own words, define each term and check your definitions with the ones given in the textbook. Page references to the textbook are provided for each term. As you check your answers, practice the pronunciation of each term. Because the life of a patient may depend on your ability to communicate with the other members of the emergency care team, correct pronunciation is essential. Once you have checked the assigned terms, go over your own list of terms gathered during your reading of the textbook chapter. Make certain that you know the meaning and pronunciation of each term. If you believe that a term will not stay with you beyond the course, consider what other words you can use to relate information to EMTs and other personnel in the EMS system. Remember, they are trained to take your information and to help you report what you have gained from interviewing, examining, and providing care for a patient.

Step 4. The fourth step is to begin the exercises. These will take the form of completions, labeling, listing, matching, chart completion, and short essays. Do *not* look up the answers in your textbook. Try to answer each question as best you can; then go to the textbook to answer only those questions you are certain that you do not know. If you use the textbook merely to look up every answer, you will be unable to determine what material you know or don't know.

Step 5. The fifth step is to check your answers with the ones provided in the exercise answers at the back of the workbook. In some cases, you will find only page references. These are for answers that are too long to reproduce in the workbook or that relate to an illustration. Keep in mind that the wording of your answers need not be the same as the answer key. The important thing is to have the same meaning. Of course, if a procedure is called for in a step-by-step fashion, you should have your answers in the correct order. Should you find one of your answers to be incorrect, use the textbook reference provided in the answer key so that you may restudy the specific information in the chapter.

Step 6. Once you have all the correct answers for the exercises in each module's chapter(s), take the module review. However, it is recommended that you let some time pass between the exercises and the review self-test. If you wait at least an hour (a whole day would be ideal), then you can test yourself to see whether you are retaining the material. A self-test is just that. It allows you to test yourself before you have to take a quiz or test in the classroom. Complete the entire review without stopping to use your notes or the textbook to find the answers.

Step 7. After completing a module review, you should check your answers with the ones provided in the module review answers at the back of the workbook. If you have an incorrect answer, you can use the textbook page reference provided to look up the materials you need to restudy.

Step 8. The final step is to go back to the textbook and use the list of objectives for each chapter in a module. Study the objectives as if they were questions and exercises. See whether you can define, list, describe, relate, label, and so on, as called for by the objectives. If your instructor has given you additional objectives, do the same for them.

This edition of the workbook offers several features—Personal Development, Application, and Additional Resources. It is a personal choice or that of your instructor as to when to complete each activity. Perhaps the best time to begin the Personal Development and Application activities is after Step 5; however; you may wish to wait until after Step 6 or Step 7. In some cases, setting aside time for these activities may have to wait until after your course. The Personal Development and Application sections will help you to reinforce your learning of Emergency Medical Responder concepts and procedures. Basically, the activities help the beginning Emergency Medical Responder develop professionalism. The Application scenarios help you bring together the various aspects of assessment-based Emergency Medical Responder-level emergency care. Some of these problems have challenged Emergency Medical Responder students during the last 15 years of program development. These problems may be part of a formal lesson in the classroom or assigned for you to complete on your own or as a member of a small group. You and your fellow students may wish to create additional situations to help you prepare for your final exam and practical. The Additional Resources section at the end of each chapter provides a listing of materials that will assist you in finding out more about the topics in each chapter.

You may be surprised to find that your workbook contains answers to the exercises. This has been done for several reasons. First of all, in most courses, instructors will not have time to collect and check every exercise done by every student. Even if they did, they would not have time to go over each wrong answer and show you where the correct information was given in the textbook. Second, most Emergency Medical Responder courses are too short for the instructor to take up class and lab time going over each exercise to give you the correct answer: The class time for workbook exercises can be better spent by going over those questions that many of the students found to be difficult. The third reason is the major one. You are an adult taking a continuing education course. You know that using the answer key to complete the exercises will not help you learn or find your own weaknesses. If you opt not to do your own work on the exercises, classroom testing will spot your weaknesses and take points away from your effort to pass the course.

Some students, and a few instructors, find the concept of self-tests difficult to understand. They ask, "What questions can be asked in classroom testing after doing the self-test?" Well, in some cases, the same questions. Perhaps they will be reworded or put into different form such as matching or labeling. Other classroom exam questions may be from rewording the chapter objectives (thus the importance of Step 8). Educational research in the last decade has shown that students need to know what is expected of them and they need to be able to monitor their own progress. Objectives, self-instructional exercises, and self-tests combine to help provide for these needs. Otherwise, a student who needs to develop organizational skills does poorly at the beginning of a course, even though he may know more than other students. Also, a student needing practice at taking tests may do poorly whereas a "next-smart" student knowing less information may do better in the course. The format of self-instruction and evaluation has proven to be the most significant in the case of an adult learner.

The last activity in the workbook is a posttest to help you prepare for your course final or state examination. Your instructor may wish to have you skip certain questions that do not apply to your specific course.

He or she may also wish to add questions to the ones provided in this workbook. Even though a "generic" posttest cannot be expected to cover all aspects of your Emergency Medical Responder course, various forms of this particular posttest have proven to be helpful to many students over the last two decades. Good luck preparing for your final exam.

So, the responsibility for learning is now yours. The textbook, the workbook, and your instructor will help you to learn. It is hoped that your study to become an Emergency Medical Responder will be both enjoyable and fascinating, leaving you with the desire to know even more and the confidence to provide Emergency Medical Responder-level emergency care. The authors welcome not only your comments on the textbook and workbook, but also any comments you may have in general about learning to be an Emergency Medical Responder.

ACKNOWLEDGMENTS

The Emergency Medical Responder Workbook begins its 8th edition, having proven itself in previous editions to be the ideal blend of knowledge and application for several hundred thousand Emergency Medical Responder students. As the program of study changes so too have the textbook and workbook. This would not have been possible without the help of many publishing and Emergency Medical Services (EMS) experts.

In particular, let me thank my new coauthor for both the textbook and this workbook, Chris Le Baudour. Chris has worked continuously in EMS since 1978, serving as an EMT-I and EMT-II in both field and clinical settings in California. In 1984, Chris began his teaching career in the California Department of Public Safety—EMS Division at Santa Rosa Junior College in Santa Rosa. He is known as an innovative instructor of Emergency Medical Technicians and Emergency Medical Responders in California's EMS system and workplace-based Emergency Medical Responder programs. At the national level, Chris serves on the Board of Directors of the National Association of EMS Educators and travels the nation speaking at EMS conferences.

Contributions to past editions continue to influence this new edition or have served as a foundation for its exercises and activities. We wish to thank Gloria Bizjak of the Maryland Fire and Rescue Institute at the University of Maryland, College Park, Maryland, for her participation on the textbook and past editions of the workbook, helping to create and extend the history of the workbook's pedagogical strengths. Gloria's unique offering of instructional methods served to help the authors of this workbook introduce a variety of learning tools and practice situations for today's Emergency Medical Responder student. Additionally, along with Gloria and myself, Bill Krause's work in the 6th edition of the textbook carries over into this edition of the workbook with the flow-of-care diagrams, which he helped us bring into the teaching methodologies offered to students learning Emergency Medical Responder-level assessment and care.

In addition to those mentioned above, we wish to thank some very gifted members of the EMS community for their reviews during various stages of the development of the seventh edition manuscript. These professionals include:

Ehren Ngo
Loma Linda University
Loma Linda, California

Francis Stewart-Dore
Southern Maine Community College
South Portland, Maine

Charles Morris
North Mississippi EMS
Nettleton, Mississippi

The authors would also like to thank the people at Prentice Hall who participated in marketing, editorial, art, and production. Quality is due to the efforts of all these individuals.

J. David Bergeron
Chris Le Baudour

Introduction to EMS Systems

Reading Assignment: First Responder, 8th Edition, pages 1–19

KEY TERMS & DEFINITIONS

Define the following terms from Chapter 1. Textbook page references are provided so that you can check your answers.

1. Emergency Medical Services system. (p. 4)

   _____

   _____

2. Medical Direction (offline & online) (pp. 8–9)

   _____

   _____

3. Scope of Practice. (p. 9)

   _____

   _____

4. Protocols. (p. 8)

   _____

   _____

5. Standing Orders. (pp. 8–9)

   _____

   _____

EXERCISES

Complete the following exercises. Answers and/or textbook page references are provided at the back of the workbook. Before looking up your answers, think about your responses and discuss them with other students, Emergency Medical Responders, and emergency care providers.

© 2009 by Pearson Education, Inc. *First Responder*, Eighth Edition, Bergeron et al.

THE EMS SYSTEM

1. Explain how Emergency Medical Responder training strengthens the links in the EMS system.

   _____

   _____

   _____

2. List the primary skills that Emergency Medical Responders are trained to perform.

   _____

   _____

   _____

   _____

3. Where in your region are Emergency Medical Responders most likely to be found working?

   _____

   _____

THE EMERGENCY MEDICAL RESPONDER

4. Your primary concern as an Emergency Medical Responder at an emergency scene is _____.
   Explain why.

   _____

   _____

5. The SIX major duties of an Emergency Medical Responder at an emergency scene are:
   A. _____
   B. _____
   C. _____
   D. _____
   E. _____
   F. _____

6. List SIX desirable traits of an Emergency Medical Responder.
   A. _____
   B. _____
   C. _____
   D. _____
   E. _____
   F. _____

7. List the four levels of training in a typical EMS system.

_____

_____

_____

_____

8. Describe what it means to be a patient advocate.

_____

_____

PERSONAL DEVELOPMENT

Consider what it will be like to be an Emergency Medical Responder and a member of the EMS system.

1. How will you feel if you are called upon to assess and provide care for a patient who is the victim of a serious illness or injury? How will you prepare for such an incident?

_____

_____

_____

_____

_____

_____

2. Compare your answers with your fellow students. How did your answers differ from those of your fellow students? What factors most affected your answers and those of your fellow students?

_____

_____

_____

_____

APPLICATION

You have completed your Emergency Medical Responder training. One evening while driving home from work, you come upon a vehicle that has skidded off the road and collided with a tree. You pull safely off the side of the road, call 911 from your cellular telephone, and proceed to assist the injured occupants.

1. What agency answers the 911 calls in your area? Is this agency different from the one that would answer calls from cellular phones?

_____

_____

© 2009 by Pearson Education, Inc. *First Responder,* Eighth Edition, Bergeron et al.

2. What agencies can you expect to arrive at the scene following your call for help? What level of medical training will these individuals likely have?

_____

_____

_____

_____

_____

3. Do Emergency Medical Responders in your area carry and use Automated External Defibrillators (AEDs)? If so, which agencies carry them?

_____

_____

Discuss this case with your classmates and compare answers. If you and your classmates disagree on any answers, discuss them with your instructor.

ADDITIONAL RESOURCES

You may choose to learn more about topics included in this chapter. The following resources contain additional information on various aspects of emergency medical care:

First Responder 8th Ed. Companion Website

First Responder 8th Ed. Student CD-ROM

Emergency Medical Services Magazine

Journal of Emergency Medical Services

Legal and Ethical Issues

Reading Assignment: First Responder, 8th Edition, pages 20–36

KEY TERMS & DEFINITIONS

Define and explain the following terms from Chapter 2. Textbook page references are provided so that you can check your answers.

1. Define the term **consent** and list the various types of consent. (pp. 24–26)

   _____

   _____

   _____

2. Define the term **abandonment** and give an example of how it may occur (pp. 29–30)

   _____

   _____

   _____

3. Explain the concept of **competence** and how it relates to patient care. (p. 24)

   _____

   _____

   _____

4. What is **refusal of care**, and when does a patient have the right to refuse care? (pp. 24–25)

   _____

   _____

   _____

5. Define **duty to act** and explain its relationship to **negligence**. (pp. 28–29)

   _____

   _____

   _____

EXERCISES

Complete the following exercises. Answers and/or textbook page references are provided at the back of the workbook. Before looking up your answers, think about your responses and discuss them with other students, Emergency Medical Responders, and emergency care providers.

SCOPE OF PRACTICE AND CONSENT

1. Explain the difference between the terms "scope of practice" and "standard of care."

   _____

   _____

   _____

2. List the Emergency Medical Responder's ethical responsibilities. Why do you think they are important?

   _____

   _____

3. List three things you should do if a patient refuses care.

   _____

   _____

   _____

4. Match the following types of consent with their explanations.

   _____ 1. Expressed consent
   _____ 2. Informed consent
   _____ 3. Implied consent
   _____ 4. Minor consent

   A. Explaining the risks/benefits of care to the patient.

   B. An unresponsive patient is assumed to want help.

   C. The patient provides verbal permission to provide care.

   D. Caring for a child in the absence of a parent.

5. A family calls for help for a family member who has a do not resuscitate (DNR) order. In what form can a DNR order be presented? Under what circumstances might you still begin resuscitation even if the family states the patient has a DNR order?

   _____

   _____

   _____

NEGLIGENCE AND ABANDONMENT

6. When does an Emergency Medical Responder have a duty to act?

   _____

   _____

© 2009 by Pearson Education, Inc. *First Responder*, Eighth Edition, Bergeron et al.

7. List the FOUR key elements of a successful negligence lawsuit.

_____

_____

_____

_____

8. Explain the purpose of Good Samaritan laws and who they are designed to protect.

_____

_____

9. Once you have started patient care, what conditions must be met before you may discontinue caring for the patient?

_____

_____

_____

CONFIDENTIALITY AND SPECIAL SITUATIONS

10. Emergency Medical Responders are restricted by law as to with whom they may share specifics about a patient's medical condition or the care that was provided. Under what circumstances can an Emergency Medical Responder share confidential patient information and with whom may they share it?

_____

_____

11. Patient confidentiality does not apply if you are required by law to report certain incidents. These incidents include:

_____

_____

12. Is emergency care for a patient who is an organ donor the same as emergency care for a patient who is not a donor? Explain your answer.

_____

_____

13. Explain an Emergency Medical Responder's priorities after police have secured a crime scene.

_____

_____

14. Explain why record keeping, or documentation, is an important part of patient care.

_____

_____

PERSONAL DEVELOPMENT

Consider the moral and ethical aspects of being an Emergency Medical Responder. Think about the standard of care in your area. How does your duty to act differ when on duty as an Emergency Medical Responder as opposed to being off duty? How will you uphold the standard and protect yourself from a lawsuit? Will you worry about being sued?

_____

_____

_____

_____

_____

_____

_____

APPLICATION

You are working as an Emergency Medical Responder for a local fire department when you are dispatched for a "man down" behind the theater. Upon arrival you find an approximately 15-year-old male lying unresponsive on the ground. Your assessment reveals that he is breathing adequately and has a strong regular pulse. You initiate care of an open wound on his right arm when he becomes responsive and refuses your efforts to assist. Describe your approach and care for this patient by answering the following questions:

1. Based on what type of consent are you allowed to care for this patient while he is unresponsive?

   _____

2. Once he becomes responsive, does the patient have the legal right to refuse care?

   _____

3. What are your options regarding care for this patient?

   _____

   _____

Discuss this case with your classmates and compare answers. If you and your classmates disagree on any answers, discuss them with your instructor. In addition, discuss the rules in your state regarding minors and consent.

ADDITIONAL RESOURCES

You may choose to learn more about topics included in this chapter. The following reference may be helpful:

Lazar, Richard. *EMS Law*. Rockville, MD: Aspen.

Contact your local or state EMS agency office for specifics on laws and regulations in your area.

Well-Being of the Emergency Medical Responder

Reading Assignment: First Responder, 8th Edition, pages 37–57

© 2009 by Pearson Education, Inc. *First Responder*, Eighth Edition, Bergeron et al.

KEY TERMS & DEFINITIONS

Define and explain the following terms from Chapter 3. Textbook page references are provided so that you can check your answers.

1. Describe each of the five stages of the grieving process listed below from the patient's perspective. (p. 39)

   Denial _____

   Anger _____

   Bargaining _____

   Depression _____

   Acceptance _____

2. From your own experience, what is your definition of **stress**? What signs and symptoms will stress produce in you? (p. 40)

   _____

   _____

3. Define the term **critical incident stress debriefing (CISD)** and explain when a CISD is typically conducted. (p. 45)

   _____

4. Describe the concept of **body substance isolation** precautions and the importance of BSI to the Emergency Medical Responder's safety. (pp. 46–47)

   _____

   _____

5. Describe the term **pathogen** and its role in the transmission of disease. (p. 48)

_____

_____

6. What is **human immunodeficiency virus (HIV)** and how can Emergency Medical Responders protect themselves from it? (p. 49)

_____

7. What is **hepatitis B** and how is it different from HIV? (p. 49)

_____

8. Describe **tuberculosis** and how Emergency Medical Responders should protect themselves from it. (pp. 49–51)

_____

9. Describe **meningitis** and how it is transmitted. (p. 51)

_____

_____

EXERCISES

Complete the following exercises. Answers and/or textbook page references are provided at the back of the workbook. Before looking up your answers, think about your responses and discuss them with other students, Emergency Medical Responders, and emergency care providers.

EMOTIONAL ASPECTS OF EMERGENCY MEDICAL CARE

1. List FIVE approaches an Emergency Medical Responder may use when dealing with grieving patients or families.

   A. _____

   B. _____

   C. _____

   D. _____

   E. _____

2. List FIVE signs and symptoms of stress.

   A. _____

   B. _____

   C. _____

   D. _____

   E. _____

3. List THREE ways of changing your lifestyle that will help you deal with stress.

A. _____

B. _____

C. _____

BODY SUBSTANCE ISOLATION (BSI)

4. What is a major safety concern of Emergency Medical Responders who must provide emergency care for victims who are ill or injured?

_____

_____

5. For which patients should the Emergency Medical Responder consider using BSI precautions?

_____

_____

6. Complete the following chart by listing FOUR pieces of personal protective equipment and explaining when the items should be worn.

PPE item	Should Be Worn During

SCENE SAFETY

7. Explain why it is important for you to do a scene size-up before approaching the patient.

_____

_____

8. Match the following situations, which may pose an increased risk to the Emergency Medical Responder, with the actions you might take to minimize exposure.

_____ 1. Hazardous Materials Incidents

_____ 2. Crime Scenes

_____ 3. Rescue Operations

A. PPE may include turnout gear and helmet.

B. Use the *Emergency Response Guidebook*.

C. It will be necessary to wait until law enforcement arrives to make it safe for you to perform your duties.

© 2009 by Pearson Education, Inc. *First Responder*, Eighth Edition, Bergeron et al.

PERSONAL DEVELOPMENT

Consider how you might feel if you were asked to care for a patient who has an infectious disease. Will you do anything differently while providing care because you know the infectious status of the patient?

_____

_____

_____

_____

_____

_____

APPLICATION

You have just transferred care of an approximately 30-year-old homeless assault victim to the ambulance crew. Before caring for the patient you donned protective gloves and eyeglasses; however, while caring for his head wound you got a moderate amount of blood on your gloved hands. Later that day the ambulance crew called your station to inform you that the patient tested positive for hepatitis B.

1. How is hepatitis B transmitted, and can it be passed through protective gloves?

   _____

   _____

2. Would you have done anything different in terms of your own protection had you known he was HBV positive?

   _____

   _____

3. What would you do if you had no personal protective equipment?

   _____

   _____

Discuss this case with your classmates and compare answers. If you and your classmates disagree on any answers, discuss them with your instructor.

ADDITIONAL RESOURCES

You may choose to learn more about topics included in this chapter. The following references may be helpful:

Emergency Response Guidebook. U.S. Department of Transportation.

The Occupational Safety and Health Administration (OSHA) publishes various documents and guidelines on infectious disease, prevention, and personal protective equipment.

The Occupational Safety and Health Administration at http://www.osha.gov

Centers for Disease Control and Prevention at http://www.cdc.gov

The Human Body

Reading Assignment: First Responder, 8th Edition, pages 58–81

KEY TERMS & DEFINITIONS

Define and explain the following terms from Chapter 4. Textbook page references are provided so that you can check your answers.

1. Describe the **anatomical position** and explain its usefulness to the Emergency Medical Responder. (p. 60)

    _____

    _____

2. Define the following terms and list an example of how each term can be used. (p. 61)

    anterior _____

    _____

    posterior _____

    _____

    medial _____

    _____

    lateral _____

    _____

    proximal _____

    _____

    distal _____

    _____

3. **Superior** means _____, whereas **inferior** means _____. (p. 61)

4. What is the **thoracic cavity?** List the organs that it contains. (p. 64)

    _____

    _____

5. Describe the function of the **diaphragm** and explain its location within the body. (p. 64)

_____

_____

EXERCISES

Complete the following exercises. Answers and/or textbook page references are provided at the back of the workbook. Before looking up your answers, think about your responses and discuss them with other students, Emergency Medical Responders, and emergency care providers.

OVERVIEW OF THE HUMAN BODY

1. Use the following terms to label Figure 4.1.

anterior	medial	distal
posterior	midline	right
superior	lateral	left
inferior	proximal	

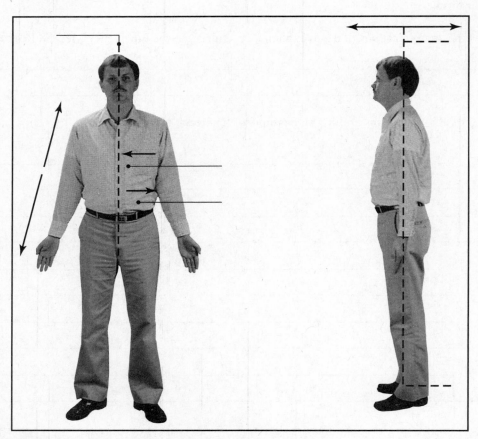

Figure 4.1 Directional terms.

2. List the parts of the upper extremity.

_____

_____

3. Label the body cavities in Figure 4.2.

© 2009 by Pearson Education, Inc. *First Responder*, Eighth Edition, Bergeron et al.

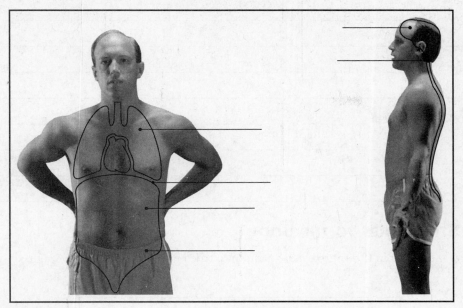

Figure 4.2 Body cavities.

4. Name two structures found in each of the abdominal quadrants. Do NOT list the small intestine or use the large intestine more than once.

RUQ	LUQ
RLQ	LLQ

BODY SYSTEMS

5. State the major function(s) of each of the following body systems:

Circulatory System _____

_____

Respiratory System _____

_____

Digestive System _____

_____

Urinary System _____

_____

Reproductive System _____

_____

© 2009 by Pearson Education, Inc. *First Responder*, Eighth Edition, Bergeron et al.

Nervous System _____

_____

Endocrine System _____

_____

Musculoskeletal System _____

_____

Special Senses _____

_____

RELATING STRUCTURES TO THE BODY

6. On Figure 4.3, draw in the approximate position of the heart, lungs, and diaphragm.

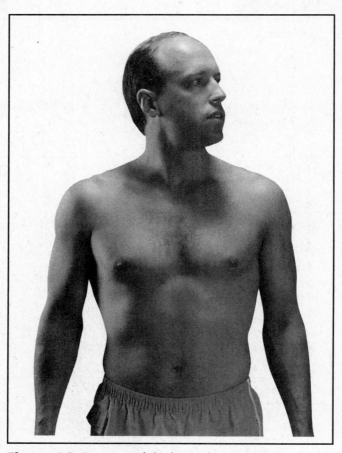

Figure 4.3 Position of the heart, lungs, and diaphragm.

7. On the photo at the left in Figure 4.4, draw the approximate position of the stomach. On the photo at the right, draw the approximate position of the liver.

8. On the photo at the left in Figure 4.5, indicate the approximate position of the small intestine. On the photo at the right, draw the approximate position of the large intestine.

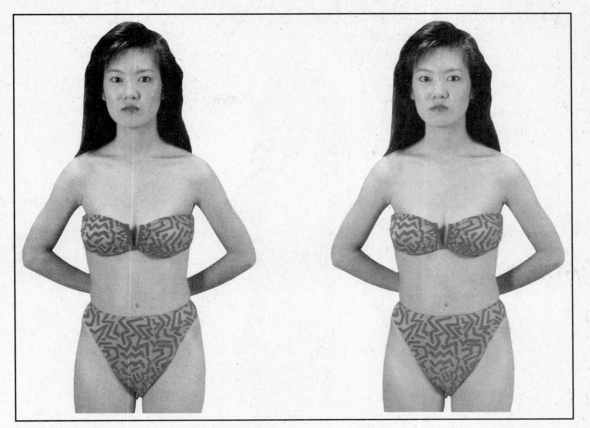

Figure 4.4 The stomach, duodenum, and liver.

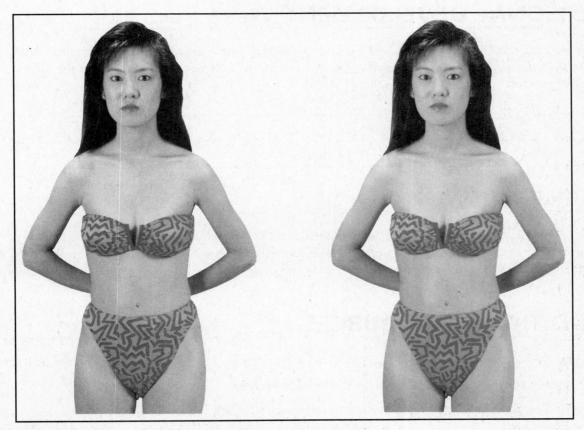

Figure 4.5 The small and large intestine.

9. On Figure 4.6, draw the approximate position of the kidneys, ureters, and urinary bladder.

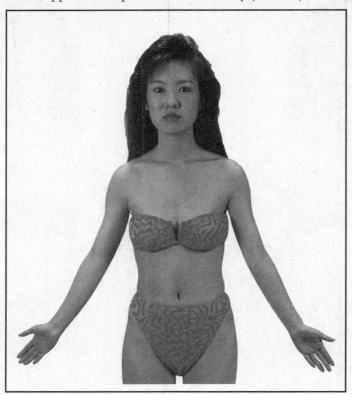

Figure 4.6 The kidneys, ureters, and urinary bladder.

PERSONAL DEVELOPMENT

Since studying this chapter, how has your view of the human body changed in terms of what you know about the body's contents, positioning of organs, and its overall complexity? What areas of the body do you feel are most vulnerable to injury and why?

_____

_____

APPLICATION

Thus far, you have learned about the human body by reading and filling in several diagrams. Now, try applying your knowledge to real-life situations. Perform patient assessments on family members and friends of different sizes and ages. Visualize and feel organs and bones as you palpate. What are your "patients'" reactions and questions?

ADDITIONAL RESOURCES

You may choose to learn more about topics included in this chapter. The following references may be helpful:

Gray's *Anatomy Coloring Book*. Philadelphia, PA: Running Press.

Fremgen, Bonnie F., PhD. *Medical Terminology*. Upper Saddle River, NJ: Brady/Prentice Hall.

Emergency Medical Update—Autopsy Video Series.

Lifting, Moving, and Positioning Patients

Reading Assignment: First Responder, 8th Edition, pages 82–109

KEY TERMS & DEFINITIONS

Define and explain the following terms from Chapter 5. Textbook page references are provided so that you can check your answers.

1. Define the term **body mechanics.** Explain why Emergency Medical Responders should use proper body mechanics to lift and move patients. (pp. 84–85)

    _____

    _____

    _____

    _____

    _____

2. Define the term **emergency move.** When will Emergency Medical Responders use emergency moves? (p. 86)

    _____

    _____

    _____

    _____

3. Define the term **nonemergency move.** When will Emergency Medical Responders use nonemergency moves? (p. 88)

    _____

    _____

    _____

    _____

© 2009 by Pearson Education, Inc. *First Responder*, Eighth Edition, Bergeron et al.

4. Discuss the importance of the **recovery position** as well as the indications and contraindications for placing a patient in this position. (pp. 94–95)

_____

_____

_____

_____

_____

EXERCISES

Complete the following exercises. Answers and/or textbook page references are provided at the back of the workbook. Before looking up your answers, think about your responses and discuss them with other students, Emergency Medical Responders, and emergency care providers.

BODY MECHANICS AND LIFTING TECHNIQUES

1. List SIX rules pertaining to safety that must be followed when lifting a patient.

    A. _____

    B. _____

    C. _____

    D. _____

    E. _____

    F. _____

MOVING AND POSITIONING PATIENTS

2. List SIX patient conditions that would be criteria for a nonemergency move.

    A. _____

    B. _____

    C. _____

    D. _____

    E. _____

    F. _____

3. Classify each of the following moves as either:

    E = Emergency move

    N = Nonemergency move

    _____ A. Firefighter's carry

    _____ B. Pack strap carry

    _____ C. Extremity lift

© 2009 by Pearson Education, Inc. *First Responder,* Eighth Edition, Bergeron et al.

_____ D. One-rescuer drag

_____ E. Direct ground lift

4. Name FOUR one-rescuer drags.

_____   _____

_____   _____

When would you use a one-rescuer drag?

_____

_____

5. Which emergency move is recommended for the patient who can walk on his own?

_____

6. In what bodily direction should you drag a patient who has a suspected spinal injury? Why?

_____

_____

7. Describe the positions of the three rescuers in the direct ground lift of the patient with no spinal injuries.

Rescuer 1 _____

Rescuer 2 _____

Rescuer 3 _____

EQUIPMENT FAMILIARITY

8. Fill in the following chart of typical carrying and packaging devices.

Type of Device	Situations in which the device would be used
Wheeled Stretcher	
Portable Stretcher	
Stair Chair	
Scoop Stretcher	
Long Spine Board	
Short Spine Board	
Vest-Type Extrication Device	
Basket Stretcher (Stokes)	
Flexible Stretcher	

© 2009 by Pearson Education, Inc. *First Responder*, Eighth Edition, Bergeron et al.

PERSONAL DEVELOPMENT

Each of us has limitations in our ability to perform certain physical tasks. List yours as they apply to moving patients. Next, use this information to describe the best positioning for you in multiple-rescuer moves. Finally, state what you need to do to improve your ability to help move patients.

_____

_____

_____

_____

_____

_____

_____

APPLICATION

You and another Emergency Medical Responder are caring for a patient who has fallen approximately 12 feet from a roof onto a hard surface. He is lying face down when you arrive on the scene. Based on the mechanism of injury, you suspect the patient may have a neck or back injury. He has no obvious injuries or signs of trauma. Describe your approach and care for this patient by answering the following questions:

A. What is your primary concern with this patient?

_____

_____

B. Under what circumstances would you want to immediately roll this patient over? Describe how you would do this.

_____

_____

C. Under what circumstances, if any, would you leave this patient face down?

_____

_____

Discuss this case with your classmates and compare your answers. If you and your classmates disagree on any answers, discuss them with your instructor.

ADDITIONAL RESOURCES

You may choose to learn more about topics included in this chapter. The following reference may be helpful:

"EMT-Free." Video about lifting and moving techniques with EMT back care in mind. Ferno–Washington, Inc., 70 Weil Way, Wilmington, OH 45177.

© 2009 by Pearson Education, Inc. _First Responder,_ Eighth Edition, Bergeron et al.

MODULE 1 REVIEW

This self-test has been designed for you to take after you have completed the Reading Assignment, Key Terms & Definitions, and Exercises for Chapters 1–5. The answers and page references are given at the end of the workbook.

CIRCLE the letter of the correct answer to each question.

1. The complete chain of professionals and services linked together to provide emergency care is the:
   - A. rescue squad.
   - B. EMS system.
   - C. life support system.
   - D. DOT.

2. The person who maintains oversight of the patient care aspects of the EMS system is known as the:
   - A. Emergency Medical Responder.
   - B. dispatcher.
   - C. Medical Director.
   - D. paramedic.

3. The primary concern of an Emergency Medical Responder at an emergency is:
   - A. traffic control.
   - B. patient care.
   - C. personal safety.
   - D. patient assessment.

4. Which of the following is one of the four main duties of an Emergency Medical Responder at the scene of an emergency?
   - A. rapidly transporting a patient to the hospital
   - B. explaining patient care details to bystanders
   - C. ensuring other units are en route before starting care
   - D. providing emergency care using minimal equipment

5. An injured patient asks if he is hurt. Which of the following responses would be most appropriate?
   - A. You are okay. Just relax and let us take care of everything.
   - B. Don't worry, everything is all right.
   - C. Could be a lot worse, you could have broken something.
   - D. We will do everything we can to see that you are cared for properly.

6. After responding to several serious incidents in a relatively short period of time, an Emergency Medical Responder is trying to deal with his stress. Which of the following is often helpful when dealing with stress from a critical incident?
   - A. emotional crisis care
   - B. critical incident stress debriefing
   - C. periodic debriefing
   - D. violence-control training

7. While responding to a multivehicle collision on the interstate, the Emergency Medical Responders are donning gloves and ensuring they have masks and eye protection readily available. With this equipment, they are:
   - A. guaranteeing personal safety.
   - B. avoiding patient contact.
   - C. providing a false sense of security.
   - D. taking body substance isolation precautions.

8. The disease that causes the greatest number of deaths among health care workers is:
   - A. HIV (AIDS).
   - B. hepatitis B.
   - C. tuberculosis.
   - D. meningitis.

© 2009 by Pearson Education, Inc. *First Responder*, Eighth Edition, Bergeron et al.

9. Which of the following diseases can be transmitted by airborne droplets?

   A. HIV (AIDS)
   B. hepatitis

   C. hepatitis and tuberculosis
   D. tuberculosis and meningitis

10. The disease that causes an inflammation of the lining of the brain and spinal cord is:

    A. HIV (AIDS).
    B. hepatitis.

    C. tuberculosis.
    D. meningitis.

11. An OSHA-mandated infectious disease program includes:

    A. a free hepatitis B vaccination and training in the use of personal protective equipment.
    B. optional pre exposure follow-up.
    C. mandatory blood tests for HIV infection.
    D. reasonable costs for purchasing protective equipment.

12. Which of the following allows an Emergency Medical Responder's actions to be judged based on what is expected of someone with his training and experience?

    A. Medical Practices Act
    B. Standard of care

    C. Implied consent laws
    D. Good Samaritan laws

13. When caring for a responsive adult patient who answers your questions in a manner that indicates he is of clear mind but refuses your care, you should:

    A. provide care anyway and make certain that the EMS system has been alerted.
    B. not provide care but tell him to call his physician.
    C. stay with the patient while waiting for EMS to arrive.
    D. provide care under the guidelines of implied consent.

14. Before providing care for a consenting adult, you should tell the patient:

    A. that treatment involves risks.
    B. what the postcare outcome will be.
    C. what you are going to do.
    D. that everything is going to be okay.

15. You believe that an injured patient in need of immediate basic emergency care is severely mentally retarded. You cannot contact his legal guardian. You should:

    A. provide care under the guidelines of implied consent.
    B. wait for the next level of care providers to arrive at the scene.
    C. not provide care if the patient says not to.
    D. not provide care until the legal guardian can be reached.

16. Do Not Resuscitate orders are advance directives that:

    A. can be ignored if the patient becomes unconscious.
    B. are mandatory for hospice or terminally ill patients
    C. may be in the form of a medical identity bracelet.
    D. will require witnesses if resuscitation is not performed.

17. An Emergency Medical Responder's best protection from a lawsuit is to:

    A. rely on the Good Samaritan law for legal protection.
    B. rely on a strong legal defense team.
    C. provide care consistent with the local standard of care.
    D. provide whatever care is necessary to save a life.

18. Good Samaritan laws may be used as legal protection:

    A. against criminal charges.
    B. in every state.
    C. if you act in good faith to provide care to the level of your training.
    D. only if you are on duty as an Emergency Medical Responder.

19. Once you have begun care, if you leave the scene before turning care over to someone of equal or greater training, you may be guilty of:

    A. abandonment.
    B. violations of the Implied Consent Act.
    C. the Medical Practices Act.
    D. a federal offense, violating the DOT Act.

20. You do not need to have a patient sign a release form to pass on information about:

    A. what a patient may have said.
    B. any unusual aspects of behavior.
    C. any descriptions of personal appearance.
    D. care procedures when transferring the patient to the next level of care.

21. Unless otherwise stated, all references to body structures are made when the body is in the

    _____ position.

    A. prone
    B. supine
    C. lateral recumbent
    D. anatomical

22. Which term can be used in describing the front of the heart?

    A. anterior
    B. posterior
    C. superior
    D. inferior

23. Structure A is closer to the midline than structure B. Structure A is said to be:

    A. lateral.
    B. proximal.
    C. medial.
    D. distal.

24. The thumb is located on the _____ side of the hand.

    A. distal
    B. lateral
    C. media
    D. proximal

25. The heart is located in the _____ cavity.

    A. thoracic
    B. spinal
    C. cranial
    D. abdominal

26. The urinary bladder is located in the _____ cavity.

    A. thoracic
    B. abdominal
    C. spinal
    D. pelvic

27. The cranial cavity houses the:

    A. lungs.
    B. brain.
    C. spinal cord.
    D. diaphragm.

28. In which abdominal quadrant is most of the liver located?

    A. RUQ
    B. LUQ
    C. RLQ
    D. LLQ

© 2009 by Pearson Education, Inc. *First Responder*, Eighth Edition, Bergeron et al.

29. Label the organs in Figure 4.7.

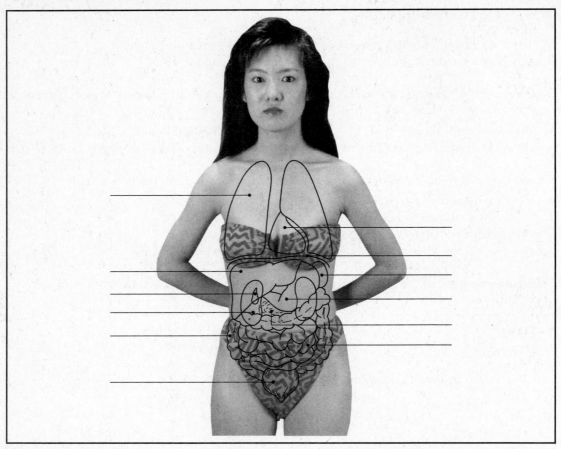

Figure 4.7 The major organs of the chest, abdomen, and pelvis.

30. When performing a one-rescuer drag, you should always drag the patient:

    A. arms first.
    B. sideways.
    C. lengthwise.
    D. feet first.

31. To perform a pack-strap carry for responsive patients, you will need:

    A. 2 rescuers.
    B. a pack strap or leather belt.
    C. a blanket.
    D. strength to carry the patient.

32. Which of the following is a requirement for a nonemergency move?

    A. The scene must be hazardous.
    B. The patient has a seriously bleeding back wound.
    C. You must reach another patient who is not breathing.
    D. The patient must be responsive.

33. What is the minimum number of rescuers recommended to perform a direct ground lift?

    A. 2
    B. 3
    C. 4
    D. 5

34. Four people have been stuck in an elevator without air conditioning for an hour. One woman faints but revives when the fire department opens the doors. She is too weak to walk and she is heavyset. What type of emergency move would you provide?
    A. extremity lift
    B. firefighter's carry
    C. blanket drag
    D. pack-strap carry

35. The most commonly used device for moving a patient, which is kept in the back of the ambulance, is the _____ stretcher.
    A. scoop
    B. flexible
    C. wheeled
    D. basket (Stokes)

Airway Management

Reading Assignment: First Responder, 8th Edition, pages 111–152

KEY TERMS & DEFINITIONS

Define and explain the following terms from Chapter 6. Textbook page references are provided so that you can check your answers.

1. Respiration. (p. 115)

   _____

   _____

   _____

2. Hypoxia. (p. 115)

   _____

   _____

   _____

3. Explain the phrase "accessory muscle use" and describe what it looks like on a patient. (p. 119)

   _____

   _____

4. Define the term **gastric distention** as it relates to rescue breathing. Describe how a patient with gastric distention might present during resuscitation. (p. 126)

   _____

   _____

   _____

   _____

5. What is the purpose of an oropharyngeal airway (OPA) and when should it be used? (pp. 138–141)

   _____

   _____

_____

_____

6. What is the function of a nasopharyngeal airway (NPA) and when should it be used? (pp. 141–142)

_____

_____

_____

_____

EXERCISES

Complete the following exercises. Answers and/or textbook page references are provided at the back of the workbook. Before looking up your answers, think about your responses and discuss them with other students, Emergency Medical Responders, and emergency care providers.

BREATHING

1. Explain the difference between clinical death and biological death.

_____

_____

_____

2. List the movement of the diaphragm muscle during inspiration and expiration. Which of these two phases is passive and which one is active?

_____

_____

_____

3. List the signs of adequate breathing.

_____

_____

_____

4. As you approach a patient, you will take the following steps to assess a patient's breathing status:

   Look for _____

   Listen for _____

   Feel for _____

5. Label the structures of the respiratory system shown in Figure 6.1.

6. List at least FIVE signs of inadequate breathing.

_____

_____

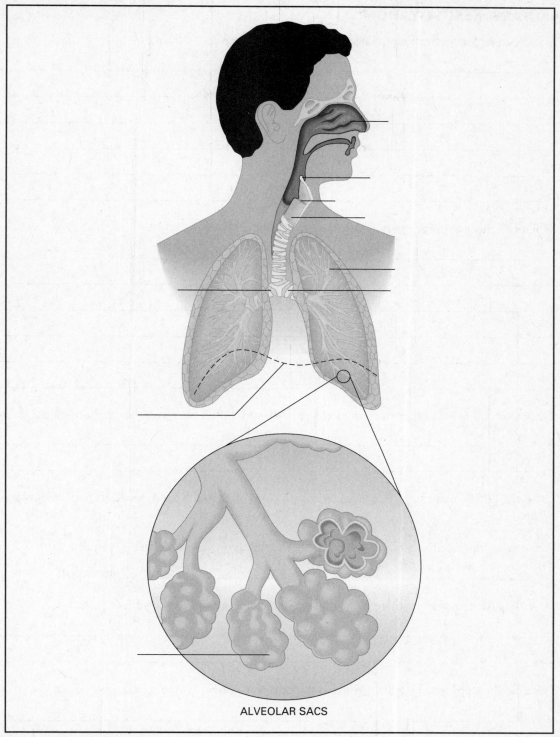

ALVEOLAR SACS

Figure 6.1 The respiratory system.

PULMONARY RESUSCITATION

7. List the steps for performing the head-tilt, chin-lift maneuver.

   _____

   _____

   _____

   _____

   _____

   _____

8. When is it most appropriate to use the jaw-thrust maneuver?

   _____

   _____

   _____

   _____

   _____

   _____

9. List at least TWO advantages of the pocket face mask with HEPA filter over the mouth-to-mouth technique.

   A. _____

   B. _____

10. Label the FOUR main steps in providing mouth-to-mask ventilation on an adult patient shown in Figure 6.2.

11. When using the mouth-to-mask technique on an adult, you should deliver

    _____ breath(s) every _____ second(s).

12. Describe how to ensure you are providing adequate ventilations to the patient.

    _____

    _____

13. Describe the steps to take when providing breaths to a patient with a stoma.

    _____

    _____

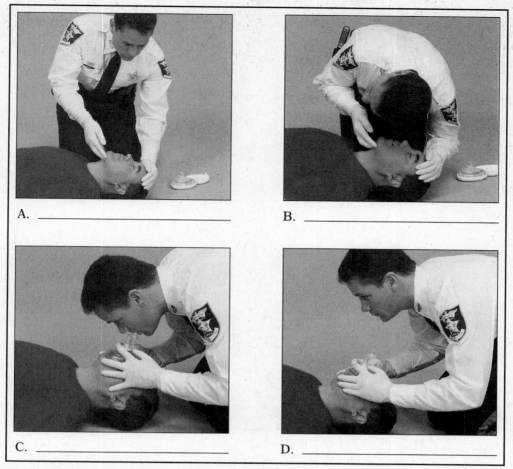

A. _____   B. _____

C. _____   D. _____

Figure 6.2 Mouth-to-mask ventilation on an adult patient.

© 2009 by Pearson Education, Inc. *First Responder*, Eighth Edition, Bergeron et al.

AIRWAY OBSTRUCTION

14. A patient with a partial airway obstruction who can produce only a very weak cough should be cared for as if he has a: _____ _____

15. List TWO signs of complete airway obstruction in the responsive patient.

_____

_____

16. Label each of the FOUR possible causes of airway obstruction shown in Figure 6.3.

17. Match the typical breathing sound to the probable partial airway obstruction.

_____ 1. Snoring

_____ 2. Gurgling

_____ 3. Crowing

_____ 4. Wheezing

A. Spasms of voice box (larynx)

B. Blood, fluids in trachea

C. Swelling or spasms along lower airway

D. Tongue obstructing back of throat

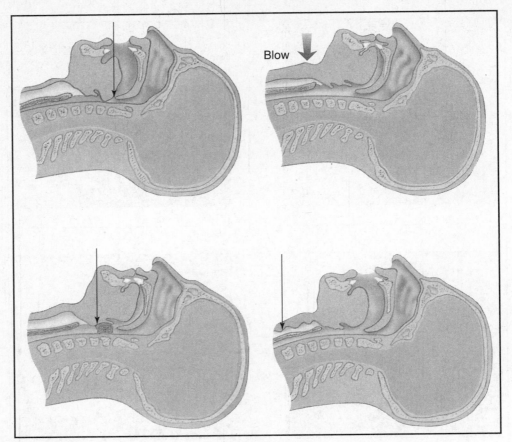

Figure 6.3 Possible causes of airway obstruction.

18. When using back blows to clear a responsive infant's airway, you should deliver up to

    _____ back blows between the shoulder blades.

19. A responsive infant has a partial airway obstruction. You note that he is NOT breathing adequately. How should you care for him?

    _____

    _____

20. When delivering abdominal thrusts to a responsive adult patient, apply rapid _____

    and _____ thrusts.

21. When delivering chest thrusts to a responsive adult patient, place one hand in a fist on the chest in the center of the sternum, between the _____.

22. _____ thrusts should be used to remove the airway obstruction of an unresponsive infant.

23. Describe how to manage a visible obstruction in the mouth of a child.

    _____

    _____

    _____

24. List the THREE main steps used to correct an airway obstruction in a responsive adult patient.

A. _____

B. _____

C. _____

25. An adult patient with a complete airway obstruction becomes unresponsive. You position the patient and open the airway. Explain what you should do next.

_____

_____

26. For a patient with an airway obstruction, you must continue to use the appropriate procedures until the airway is cleared or you have dislodged the obstruction to the point where you can provide

_____.

AIDS TO RESUSCITATION (AIRWAY ADJUNCTS)

27. The two types of airway adjuncts that may be used are the _____ airway and the _____ airway.

28. *Oro* refers to the _____, and *pharyngeo* refers to the _____. This type of airway should be used only on _____ patients who do not have a _____.

29. Describe how to measure the nasopharyngeal airway and the oropharyngeal airway.

Nasopharyngeal airway _____

_____

Oropharyngeal airway _____

_____

30. List FOUR rules of suctioning.

_____

_____

_____

PERSONAL DEVELOPMENT

Protective barriers for rescue breathing may be found in most first aid kits. Investigate this in your own community. Try your workplace, gym, or school to see if they have a protective barrier or pocket mask in the first aid kit. It is doubtful that you will find 100% availability in any community. When appropriate, always stop and check the contents of a first aid kit. Ensure that it contains the appropriate protective barriers necessary to assist an ill or injured patient. In addition to standard first aid supplies, the kit should contain protective gloves and a mouth barrier device.

APPLICATION

You are called to the scene of an approximately 60-year-old female patient who collapsed while attending church. Upon arrival you discover that she is unresponsive and not breathing adequately but has a good pulse. Bystanders have no additional information on the patient's condition or medical history. Describe your approach and care for this patient by answering the following questions:

A.   What type of body substance isolation (BSI) precautions will you use?

_____

B.   What method will you use to open the airway and why?

_____

C.   What type of airway adjunct will you use and why?

_____

D.   Because the patient is not breathing, she is in need of rescue breathing. How often will you need to breathe for this woman?

_____

Discuss this case with your classmates. Compare answers. How would you handle this situation if you had no equipment with you? What is your priority?

ADDITIONAL RESOURCES

You may choose to learn more about this topic. The following references may be helpful:

Guidelines 2005 Basic Life Support. Dallas, Texas. American Heart Association.

American Heart Association—"Currents" publication: http://www.americanheart.org

MODULE 2 REVIEW

This self-test has been designed for you to take after you have completed the Reading Assignment, Key Terms & Definitions, and Exercises for Chapter 6. The answers and page references are given at the end of the workbook.

CIRCLE the letter of the correct answer to each question.

1. The moment when both heartbeat and respirations stop, a patient is referred to as:
   - A. partially dead.
   - B. biologically dead.
   - C. clinically dead.
   - D. in a coma

2. Which of the following occurs when the volume inside the chest cavity increases and the lungs expand?
   - A. compression
   - B. concussion
   - C. expiration (exhalation)
   - D. inspiration (inhalation)

3. The purpose of the epiglottis is to:
   - A. allow air to pass by the pharynx (throat).
   - B. function as the voice box.
   - C. prevent food and fluids from entering the trachea.
   - D. exchange gases and fluids.

4. Which of the following is recommended for opening the airway of a patient with possible spinal injury?
   - A. head-tilt maneuver
   - B. head-tilt, neck-lift maneuver
   - C. head-tilt, chin-lift maneuver
   - D. jaw-thrust maneuver

5. The recommended first choice for the solo rescuer for providing rescue breaths is:
   - A. mouth-to-mouth.
   - B. artificial respiration.
   - C. mouth-to-mask.
   - D. blow-by technique.

6. When positioning a pocket face mask, the base of the mask should rest:
   - A. over the bridge of the patient's nose.
   - B. under the patient's lower jaw.
   - C. between the patient's lower lip and the chin.
   - D. below the patient's chin.

7. The recommended duration of a breath delivered to an adult patient who is in respiratory arrest is approximately _____ second(s).
   - A. 1
   - B. 1.5 to 2
   - C. 3 to 5
   - D. 3.5 to 4.

8. While performing mouth-to-mask ventilations on an adult, the recommended rate is 1 breath delivered every _____ seconds.
   - A. 3–5
   - B. 5–6
   - C. 7–8
   - D. 10

9. Which of the following is the recommended rate for providing rescue breathing to an infant?
   - A. 1 breath every 3–5 seconds
   - B. 1 breath every 5–6 seconds
   - C. 2 breaths every 5 seconds
   - D. 2 breaths every 15 seconds

© 2009 by Pearson Education, Inc. *First Responder*, Eighth Edition, Bergeron et al.

10. During rescue breathing of an adult stoma patient, a breath is provided every

   _____ seconds.

   A. 2–3   C. 10
   B. 5–6   D. 12

11. During rescue breathing, some air enters the patient's stomach. The best way to minimize this problem is to:

   A. reduce the force of your ventilations. C. push in on the patient's abdomen.
   B. reposition the patient's head.   D. turn the patient on his side.

12. The most common cause of airway obstruction in the unresponsive patient is:

   A. food.   C. fluids.
   B. the tongue.   D. voice-box spasms.

13. One sign of a partial airway obstruction is gurgling. It may be caused by:

   A. swelling in the lower airway.   C. fluids in the upper airway.
   B. the tongue obstructing the throat.   D. spasms of the voice box.

14. Which of the following patients with a partial airway obstruction should be cared for as if he had a complete obstruction?

   A. patient who is unable to cough   C. patient who is able to speak in a weak voice
   B. patient who is continuing to cough   D. patient who is crying out loudly for help

15. When correcting an infant's airway obstruction with back blows, you should deliver up to

   _____ back blows in rapid succession.

   A. 3   C. 7
   B. 5   D. 9

16. For an adult patient, chest thrusts should be applied:

   A. directly below the collarbones.
   B. slightly inferior to the diaphragm.
   C. at the xiphoid process at the base of the breastbone.
   D. over the center of the breastbone.

17. Which of the following should be used on a responsive infant with a complete upper airway obstruction?

   A. abdominal thrusts   C. chest thrusts
   B. blind finger sweeps   D. back blows and chest thrusts

18. Chest thrusts are delivered to the infant using two or three fingertips that are placed along the midline of the breastbone:

   A. directly over the xiphoid process at the base of the sternum.
   B. one finger-width below an imaginary line drawn between the nipples.
   C. directly on an imaginary line drawn between the nipples.
   D. over the top of the joints where the sternum meets with the collarbones.

© 2009 by Pearson Education, Inc. *First Responder*, Eighth Edition, Bergeron et al.

19. An unresponsive infant has an airway obstruction. You have attempted two breaths without success; what should you do next?
   A. Perform five back blows.
   B. Begin chest compressions.
   C. Deliver five chest thrusts.
   D. Perform a blind finger sweep.

20. A major advantage of an airway adjunct is that:
   A. special training is not needed for its use.
   B. it does not need to be inspected or maintained.
   C. it allows for the delivery of more effective ventilations.
   D. special adjuncts quickly saturate the lungs with oxygen.

21. An oropharyngeal airway should be used on nonbreathing patients who are:
   A. unresponsive with no gag reflex.
   B. responsive with difficulty breathing.
   C. choking on an obstruction.
   D. swelling from an allergic reaction.

22. When measuring for fit, a properly sized oropharyngeal airway will extend from the center of a patient's mouth to the:
   A. tip of the tongue.
   B. angle of the lower jaw.
   C. bridge of the nose.
   D. area in front of the uvula.

23. On an adult patient, slide the tip of the oropharyngeal airway along the roof of the mouth, past the soft tissues, and then:
   A. attempt to ventilate.
   B. secure it with tape.
   C. rotate it 180 degrees.
   D. check for a gag reflex.

24. It is appropriate to use a nasopharyngeal airway on all the following patients EXCEPT:
   A. an unresponsive patient who is in cardiac arrest.
   B. an unresponsive patient suffering an asthma attack.
   C. an unresponsive patient in shock who has suffered a fractured leg.
   D. an unresponsive patient who has suffered head and facial trauma.

25. When suctioning an adult patient's airway, you should suction only for a maximum of

   _____ seconds at a time.
   A 5
   B. 10
   C. 15
   D. 20

© 2009 by Pearson Education, Inc. *First Responder,* Eighth Edition, Bergeron et al.

Assessment of the Patient

Reading Assignment: First Responder, 8th Edition, pages 153–202

KEY TERMS & DEFINITIONS

Define and explain the following terms from Chapter 7. Textbook references are provided so that you can check your answers.

1. Define and describe the term **patient assessment**. What is its purpose? (p. 157)

   _____

   _____

2. Define and describe the term **chief complaint**. (p. 169)

   _____

   _____

3. Define the terms **mechanism of injury (MOI)** and **nature of illness (NOI)**. (pp. 157, 158)

   _____

   _____

   _____

   _____

4. What is the primary purpose of the **initial assessment**? (p. 157)

   _____

   _____

5. Explain the difference between a **sign** and a **symptom**. List two examples of each. (p. 157)

   _____

   _____

   _____

6. List all five **vital signs** and their characteristics. (p. 158)

_____

_____

_____

_____

_____

7. Describe the location of the **carotid pulse** and the **radial pulse**. (p. 174)

_____

_____

EXERCISES

Complete the following exercises. Answers and/or textbook page references are provided at the back of the workbook. Before looking up your answers, think about your responses and discuss them with other students, Emergency Medical Responders, and emergency care providers.

PATIENT ASSESSMENT COMPONENTS

1. Explain the reasoning behind learning a head-to-toe approach to patient assessment.

_____

_____

_____

2. For most patients, the assessment should begin with these FOUR parts:

A. _____

B. _____

C. _____

D. _____

3. List the FIVE major components of a patient assessment.

A. _____

B. _____

C. _____

D. _____

E. _____

© 2009 by Pearson Education, Inc. _First Responder_, Eighth Edition, Bergeron et al.

4. List the THREE major concerns you should have when assessing a patient.

First Concern	
Second Concern	
Third Concern	

SCENE SIZE-UP

5. List the FIVE components of a scene size-up.

A. _____

B. _____

C. _____

D. _____

E. _____

6. List the items you should wear when body substance isolation (BSI) precautions are needed.

_____

_____

THE INITIAL ASSESSMENT

7. Explain when an initial assessment begins.

_____

_____

8. List the SIX major parts of the initial assessment.

A. _____

B. _____

C. _____

D. _____

E. _____

F. _____

9. List the "ABCs" of emergency care and describe how each is assessed.

A. _____

B. _____

C. _____

© 2009 by Pearson Education, Inc. *First Responder*, Eighth Edition, Bergeron et al.

10. To begin the initial assessment you should form a _____ impression of the patient and the environment. Explain why this step is important.

_____

_____

_____

11. A mnemonic used to classify a patient's level of consciousness is AVPU. What does each letter of the mnemonic represent?

A _____

V _____

P _____

U _____

12. To determine adequate breathing, you must

LOOK for:

_____

LISTEN for:

_____

FEEL for:

_____

13. During the initial assessment of an unresponsive patient, circulation is determined by checking for a _____ _____ on the same side of the neck that you are positioned.

14. What kind of bleeding should you check for during the initial assessment? Why?

_____

_____

15. List EIGHT high-priority conditions that would call for an immediate transport decision.

A. _____

B. _____

C. _____

D. _____

E. _____

F. _____

G. _____

H. _____

© 2009 by Pearson Education, Inc. *First Responder*, Eighth Edition, Bergeron et al.

16. Describe how to check capillary refill in an infant or a small child. What is a normal capillary refill time?

_____

_____

_____

_____

FOCUSED HISTORY AND PHYSICAL EXAM

17. Describe the main purpose of the focused history and physical exam.

_____

_____

_____

18. Describe the type of assessment you would perform for each of the following patients.

   A. Trauma patient—no significant mechanism of injury: _____

   _____

   _____

   B. Trauma patient—significant mechanism of injury: _____

   _____

   _____

   C. Unresponsive medical patient: _____

   _____

   _____

   D. Responsive medical patient: _____

   _____

   _____

19. Complete Table 7.1. Describe the components of the SAMPLE history and give an example of each.

Table 7.1 Components of the SAMPLE History

	LETTER REPRESENTS . . .	EXAMPLE
S	Signs and Symptoms	Chest pain and shortness of breath
A		
M		
P		
L		
E		

© 2009 by Pearson Education, Inc. *First Responder,* Eighth Edition, Bergeron et al.

20. List SIX questions commonly asked of bystanders at the emergency scene.

    A. _____

    B. _____

    C. _____

    D. _____

    E. _____

    F. _____

21. When you are conducting a focused history and physical exam, when would it be appropriate to stop and care for an injury you find?

    _____

    _____

    _____

22. What might cause a patient who appears to be stable to worsen rapidly?

    _____

    _____

    _____

23. List what each letter in mnemonic DCAP-BTLS stands for:

    D _____

    C _____

    A _____

    P _____

    B _____

    T _____

    L _____

    S _____

24. List what each letter in the mnemonic BP-DOC stands for:

    B _____

    P _____

    D _____

    O _____

    C _____

25. While determining the pulse rate, you should also determine the _____ and

the _____ of the beats.

26. List possible causes of the following:

Rapid, strong pulse _____

_____

Rapid, weak pulse _____

_____

Slow pulse _____

_____

No pulse _____

_____

27. Complete Table 7.2.

Table 7.2 Normal Pulse Rates

Patient	Normal Pulse Rate
Infant (under 1 year)	_____ to _____ (beats per minute)
Child (1 to 5 years)	_____ to _____ (beats per minute)
Child (5 to 12 years)	_____ to _____ (beats per minute)
Adult	_____ to _____ (beats per minute)

28. Complete Table 7.3.

Table 7.3 Normal Respiratory Rates

Patient	Normal Respiratory Rate
Adult	_____ to _____
Child (6–10 years)	_____ to _____
Child (1–5 years)	_____ to _____
Infant	_____ to _____

© 2009 by Pearson Education, Inc. *First Responder*, Eighth Edition, Bergeron et al.

29. The following are activities performed during the rapid trauma assessment (serious mechanism, unresponsive patient). They are NOT listed in the correct order. Number these activities from 1 to 22 in the order in which they are typically performed in your EMS system.

_____ A. Check the skull for deformities and depressions.

_____ B. Inspect the chest for cuts, bruises, penetrations, and impaled objects.

_____ C. Check for nerve activity and possible paralysis to the legs and feet.

_____ D. Check the cervical spine for point tenderness and deformity.

_____ E. Examine the legs and feet.

_____ F. Examine the eyes.

_____ G. Feel the pelvis for injures and suspected fractures.

_____ H. Examine the upper extremities from shoulders and clavicles to fingertips.

_____ I. Check for equal expansion of the chest.

_____ J. Inspect the abdomen for cuts, bruises, penetrations, and impaled objects.

_____ K. Feel the abdomen for tenderness.

_____ L. Examine the chest for suspected fractures.

_____ M. Feel the clavicles for tenderness and look for deformity.

_____ N. Feel the lower back for point tenderness and look for deformity.

_____ O. Check to see if the patient is a "neck breather."

_____ P. Check for distal pulse.

_____ Q. Inspect the mouth for possible airway obstructions, bleeding, or damage.

_____ R. Inspect the ears and nose for blood, clear fluid, or bloody fluid.

_____ S. Look at the inner surface of the eyelids.

_____ T. Note any obvious injury to the genital region.

_____ U. Check the scalp for cuts and bruises.

_____ V. Inspect the back surfaces of the patient for bleeding and obvious injury.

Note: Most EMS system guidelines direct the Emergency Medical Responder to begin the examination by checking the cervical spine for tenderness and deformity, provided the head is in a stable position. This approach gives the rescuer a better chance to detect neck injuries and stabilize the head and neck before continuing the assessment.

30. Describe how you would assess the circulation, sensation, and motor function of the legs of a *responsive* patient.

_____

_____

31. Describe how you would assess the circulation, sensation, and motor function of the upper extremities of an *unresponsive* patient.

_____

_____

DETAILED PHYSICAL EXAM AND ONGOING ASSESSMENT

32. Explain when the detailed physical exam is performed.

_____

_____

_____

_____

33. List the steps of an ongoing assessment. What is the purpose of this assessment?

_____

_____

_____

_____

34. List the words that are associated with the OPQRST assessment mnemonic and provide a sample question for each:

O _____

P _____

Q _____

R _____

S _____

T _____

PERSONAL DEVELOPMENT

Take this opportunity to begin a personal file of patient assessments. You can do this on 3 × 5 cards (example follows), as a computer file, or as a simple notepaper file. Start by creating the scene of a medical or trauma emergency and write out the scene size-up elements, the initial assessment results, and the focused assessment that is suitable for the situation. For each major section of each chapter in your textbook, complete a patient file or card. When you become a practicing Emergency Medical Responder, continue building files for actual patient situations.

Remember: Be certain that you maintain patient confidentiality! Do not use patient names. This file should not replace your EMS system's required records and reports.

© 2009 by Pearson Education, Inc. *First Responder*, Eighth Edition, Bergeron et al.

MEDICAL EMERGENCY	Chief Complaint: _____

TRAUMA EMERGENCY   Chief Complaint: _____

SCENE SIZE-UP _____

_____

PATIENT ASSESSMENTS
Initial _____

_____

Focused History and Physical Exam _____

_____

Detailed _____

_____

Ongoing _____

_____

APPLICATION

You have responded to a motorcycle crash with two patients who were both wearing helmets. Patient 1 is an approximately 20-year-old male who is responsive and screaming out in pain. His chief complaint is pain in his right femur, and you notice swelling and deformity. Patient 2 is an approximately 15-year-old female who is lying face down and is unresponsive; she also has an open wound to her right forearm. She has no other obvious external trauma. Answer the following questions relating to this scenario:

1. Which of these patients has the higher priority for treatment and why?

   _____

   _____

2. Which assessment path is most appropriate for each of these patients and why?

   _____

   _____

3. Will you want to roll patient 2 over? If so, why?

   _____

   _____

4. Will you want to use spinal precautions for these patients? If so, how will you do it?

   _____

   _____

Discuss this case with your instructor and classmates. Compare answers. What is your priority when dealing with a patient with a breathing problem?

_____

_____

ADDITIONAL RESOURCES

You may choose to learn more about this topic. The following references may be helpful:

Edgerly, Dennis, EMT-P. 2008. Assessing Your Assessment. (January 24), www.JEMS.com.

Mattera, Connie, RN, MS, TNS, EMT-P. 2008. How to Approach Your Patient with Care. (May 11), www.JEMS.com.

"Beyond the Basics: Patient Assessment. Why patient assessment is one of the most important skills an EMS provider can possess." *Emergency Medical Services,* July 2006.

MODULE 3 REVIEW

This self-test has been designed for you to take after you have completed the Reading Assignment, Key Terms & Definitions, and Exercises for Chapter 7. The answers and page references are given at the end of the workbook.

CIRCLE the letter of the correct answer to each question.

1. The primary purpose of the initial assessment is to:
   A. detect all injuries and illnesses.
   B. identify and correct life-threatening problems.
   C. identify and correct all illnesses and injuries.
   D. detect all life-threatening problems.

2. The best source to find out what is wrong with a responsive patient comes from the:
   A. patient.
   B. scene.
   C. mechanism of injury.
   D. parents or guardians.

3. Respiratory status, circulation, and bleeding are first addressed during the:
   A. focused history and physical exam.
   B. head-to-toe examination.
   C. initial assessment.
   D. taking of vital signs.

4. The first two steps in the initial assessment are to:
   A. form a general impression and assess mental status.
   B. ensure an open airway and assess breathing.
   C. assess breathing and circulation.
   D. assess circulation and check for bleeding.

5. When you look, listen, and feel for breathing, you are:
   A. getting a respiratory rate.
   B. deciding on the type of artificial respiration to use.
   C. assuring the patient of your skills.
   D. checking for adequate air exchange.

6. The carotid pulse can be felt on the patient's:
   A. neck.
   B. wrist.
   C. foot.
   D. temple.

7. During the initial assessment, you are looking for _____ bleeding.
   A. uncontrolled
   B. arterial
   C. venous
   D. capillary

8. A sign is:
   A. an indication of life.
   B. what the patient tells you is wrong.
   C. what you see, hear, feel, and smell when examining the patient.
   D. the patient's answer to a specific question.

9. A symptom is:

   A. an indication of life.
   B. what the patient tells you is wrong.
   C. what you see, hear, feel, and smell when examining the patient.
   D. the patient's answer to a specific question.

10. Adequate blood flow to all cells of the body is called:

    A. shock.
    B. perfusion

    C. hypoperfusion.
    D. saturation.

11. For a patient with a significant mechanism of injury, the Emergency Medical Responder should:

    A. perform a focused trauma assessment.
    B. start an ongoing assessment.

    C. perform a rapid trauma assessment.
    D. begin a detailed physical exam.

12. You should begin your assessment of an unresponsive medical patient by:

    A. taking vital signs.
    B. gathering a SAMPLE history.

    C. conducting a detailed physical exam.
    D. performing a rapid medical exam.

13. The question "What is wrong?" asks the patient about:

    A. DCAP-BTLS.
    B. the chief complaint.

    C. vital signs.
    D. capillary refill.

14. An acronym used to obtain a patient's history is:

    A. AVPU.
    B. ABC.

    C. SAMPLE
    D. DCAP-BTLS.

15. The "A" in the acronym SAMPLE stands for:

    A. arterial bleeding
    B. assessment

    C. allergies
    D. alert

16. When assessing a pulse, you must assess for:

    A. rhythm, depth, and sound.
    B. rate, strength, and rhythm.

    C. depth, sound, and force.
    D. rate and force.

17. The normal pulse rate for an adult at rest will fall between:

    A. 40 and 70
    B. 60 and 100

    C. 80 and 100
    D. 100 and 120.

18. The characteristics of respirations include:

    A. rhythm and depth.
    B. rate, depth, and ease of breathing.
    C. rhythm, force, depth, and sound.
    D. rhythm, depth, force, and ease of breathing.

19. The normal respiration rate for an adult at rest falls into a range of _____ breaths per minute.

    A. 1 to 5
    B. 5 to 12

    C. 12 to 20
    D. 20 to 24

© 2009 by Pearson Education, Inc. *First Responder*, Eighth Edition, Bergeron et al.

20. In general, respiratory rates on an adult of less than _____ breaths per minute or greater than _____ breaths per minute may indicate a serious condition.
    A. 8, 24   C. 15, 30
    B. 12, 20   D. 25, 50

21. Unequal pupils are a possible indication of:
    A. cardiac arrest.   C. bleeding.
    B. coma.   D. stroke.

22. The "S" in the OPQRST assessment mnemonic stands for:
    A. signs   C. severity
    B. symptoms   D. smell.

23. During the patient assessment, if you notice tenderness at the cervical spine, you should:
    A. stop and immobilize the patient's head and neck.
    B. check for paralysis by pinching the patient's hand.
    C. continue with the next step in the exam.
    D. immediately check the skull for deformities and depressions.

24. The purpose of the ongoing assessment is to watch for changes in the patient's condition. Monitoring these changes are called:
    A. detailing.   C. trending.
    B. critiquing.   D. monitoring.

25. During the ongoing assessment, unstable patients should be reassessed every

    _____ minutes.
    A. 5   C. 15
    B. 10   D. 20

Resuscitation and the Use of the AED

Reading Assignment: First Responder, 8th Edition, pages 203–244

KEY TERMS & DEFINITIONS

Define and explain the following terms from Chapter 8. Textbook page references are provided so that you can check your answers.

1. Define the term **cardiac arrest**. List the signs of cardiac arrest and explain how it is managed. (pp. 206–207)

   _____

   _____

   _____

   _____

2. Describe the locations of a **brachial pulse** and a **carotid pulse**. (pp. 210–211)

   _____

   _____

   _____

3. Define the term **cardiopulmonary resuscitation**. (p. 207)

   _____

   _____

   _____

   _____

4. In terms of age, how does the American Heart Association (AHA) define the following individuals? (p. 223)

   Infant _____

   Child _____

   Adult _____

© 2009 by Pearson Education, Inc. *First Responder,* Eighth Edition, Bergeron et al.

5. Define the term **external chest compressions**. (p. 208)

_____

_____

_____

6. Describe the procedure for **single-rescuer CPR** on an adult. (pp. 211–216)

_____

_____

_____

_____

_____

_____

7. Define the term **defibrillation** and explain when and why it is used. (p. 207)

_____

_____

_____

_____

_____

_____

8. Define the term **ventricular fibrillation** and how a patient who has this might present. (p. 232–233)

_____

_____

_____

_____

_____

_____

_____

EXERCISES

Complete the following exercises. Answers and/or textbook page references are provided at the back of the workbook. Before looking up your answers, think about your responses and discuss them with other students, Emergency Medical Responders, and emergency care providers.

THE CHAIN OF SURVIVAL

1. List the FOUR elements of the chain of survival.

   A. _____

   B. _____

   C. _____

   D. _____

CARDIAC ARREST AND CPR

2. List at least THREE signs of cardiac arrest.

   A. _____

   B. _____

   C. _____

3. Explain when clinical death occurs.

   _____

   _____

4. Without oxygen, brain tissues may die within _____ to

   _____ minutes.

5. By starting CPR as soon as possible, Emergency Medical Responders can prevent

   _____ by circulating oxygenated blood to _____.

6. Explain how CPR works.

   _____

   _____

   _____

   _____

7. Explain why a patient may need only ventilations and not compressions.

   _____

   _____

   _____

© 2009 by Pearson Education, Inc. *First Responder*, Eighth Edition, Bergeron et al.

THE TECHNIQUES OF CPR

8. List the SIX actions you should perform leading up to CPR.

   A. _____

   B. _____

   C. _____

   D. _____

   E. _____

   F. _____

9. List the SIX steps for performing external chest compressions.

   A. _____

   B. _____

   C. _____

   D. _____

   E. _____

   F. _____

10. List the THREE factors to consider when providing ventilations during CPR.

    A. _____

    B. _____

    C. _____

11. When performing CPR on adult patients, you should deliver compressions at a rate of

    _____ per minute and ventilations at a ratio of two breaths every

    _____ compressions.

12. Complete the following step-by-step outline for performing CPR on adults.

1	Check for unresponsiveness.
2	Position patient and yourself.
3	Open the airway by using the _____-tilt, chin-_____.
4	Check for breathing. (LOOK, LISTEN, AND _____).
5	Provide _____ slow breaths.
6	If necessary, _____ the airway.
7	Check for signs of circulation by feeling for a _____ pulse.

8	Locate the _____ site.
9	Position your _____ on the compression site.
10	Provide _____ chest compressions.
11	Provide _____ breaths every 30 compressions.

13. Complete the following step-by-step outline for providing CPR for an infant or a child.

1	Determine unresponsiveness.
2	Call for help.
3	Correctly position the patient.
4	Open the airway.
5	Check for breathing.
6	Provide two breaths (clear obstructions if necessary).
7	Check for circulation by checking for a _____ pulse on a child, _____ pulse on an infant.
8	Provide chest compressions and ventilations at the ratio of _____:2 for children and infants.
9	Call dispatch.

14. List SEVEN techniques that will help improve the effectiveness of CPR.

A. _____

B. _____

C. _____

D. _____

E. _____

F. _____

G. _____

15. Indicate whether the hand positions in Figure 8.1 are correct or incorrect. If a position is incorrect, describe what possible damage can be done.

A. _____

B. _____

C. _____

D. _____

© 2009 by Pearson Education, Inc. *First Responder*, Eighth Edition, Bergeron et al.

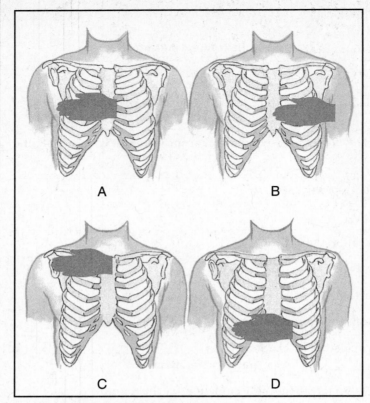

Figure 8.1 Problems during CPR.

16. List FIVE reasons for stopping CPR.

    A. _____

    B. _____

    C. _____

    D. _____

    E. _____

17. Complete Table 8.1.

Table 8.1 CPR Summary

	Compression Method	Depth (inches)	Rate (per minute)	Compressions to breaths ratio
Adult				
Child				
Infant				

18. Will defibrillation start a dead heart? Explain.

    _____

    _____

    _____

© 2009 by Pearson Education, Inc. *First Responder*, Eighth Edition, Bergeron et al.

_____

_____

_____

19. Explain why a heart in ventricular fibrillation cannot support life.

_____

_____

_____

_____

20. Answer yes or no to the following questions and briefly explain your answers. Should you defibrillate:

A. a patient who is in a moving vehicle?

_____

_____

B. a patient who has a pulse but has an obstructed airway?

_____

_____

C. a child in cardiac arrest who is 10 years of age?

_____

_____

21. In SIX steps, describe how to attach a defibrillator to a patient.

A. _____

B. _____

C. _____

D. _____

E. _____

F. _____

22. You are using an automated external defibrillator. The pads have been placed on the patient's chest and the cables are connected. No one is in contact with the patient or the device, and you have pressed the defibrillator ON button. The voice synthesizer should direct you to:

_____

_____

© 2009 by Pearson Education, Inc. *First Responder*, Eighth Edition, Bergeron et al.

23. An automated external defibrillator has delivered one shock to a patient. After this is done, the voice synthesizer should direct you to:

_____

_____

24. Most of the problems of defibrillation that can be corrected by the Emergency Medical Responder in-

volve _____ and/or _____ .

25. In the space below, diagram the proper placement of the pads of an automated external defibrillator. Then describe how to operate the defibrillator that is most commonly used in your response area.

_____

_____

_____

_____

_____

_____

_____

PERSONAL DEVELOPMENT

Many lay people believe that CPR will "bring a patient back to life." They also believe that in all cases CPR will maintain life so that the emergency department staff can use more advanced techniques to save the patient. As a member of the EMS system, you represent a source of knowledge and understanding for the lay public. Outline the way in which you would explain to a group of adults the limitations of CPR.

_____

_____

_____

_____

_____

_____

© 2009 by Pearson Education, Inc. *First Responder*, Eighth Edition, Bergeron et al.

Automated External Defibrillators (AEDs) are becoming increasingly common. In some states, legislation has made the devices easier for agencies and organizations to implement, and the average price continues to drop. As an Emergency Medical Responder, you should

. . . become familiar with AEDs within your agency or community.

. . . practice how you would use the AED in the event of an actual cardiac emergency.

APPLICATION

You have been dispatched on a call for a "man down" in the parking lot of a local convenience store. Upon arrival you find an approximately 60-year-old male lying supine on the ground. A bystander is performing chest compressions. Describe your approach and care for this patient by answering the following questions:

1. What will be the first thing you do as you approach the patient (scene is safe, BSI precautions have been taken)?

    _____

    _____

2. Will you immediately take over for the bystander? If not, why?

    _____

    _____

3. At what point will you apply the AED?

    _____

    _____

Discuss this case with your classmates and compare answers. If you and your classmates disagree on any answers, discuss them with your instructor.

ADDITIONAL RESOURCES

You may choose to learn more about this topic. The following references may be helpful:

Healthcare Provider Video. American Heart Association, Dallas, TX. A guide for Healthcare Providers who serve as Emergency Medical Responders to cardiac emergencies.

The definitive resource for Automated External Defibrillator (AED) information and technology at http://www.aed.com

MODULE 4 REVIEW

This self-test has been designed for you to take after you have completed the Reading Assignment, Key Terms & Definitions, and Exercises for Chapter 8. The answers and page references are given at the end of the workbook.

CIRCLE the letter of the correct answer to each question.

1. The most appropriate pulse to use for the unresponsive adult is the:
   A. circulation.
   B. compression.
   C. carotid pulse.
   D. cardiac arrest.

2. If respiratory arrest and cardiac arrest occur:
   A. the brain will die immediately.
   B. brain function is reduced by half.
   C. changes leading to brain cell death will soon occur.
   D. the brain will become hyperactive.

3. When assessing breathing, you should look, listen, and feel for no more than _____ seconds.
   A. 3
   B. 5
   C. 10
   D. 10 to 12

4. During CPR, compressions for the adult patient are delivered at a rate of _____ per minute.
   A. 50 to 60
   B. 60 to 80
   C. 70 to 90
   D. approximately 100

5. The depth of compressions for the adult patient is _____ inch(es).
   A. ½ to 1
   B. 1 to 1½
   C. 1½ to 2
   D. 2 to 21

6. During CPR, ventilations for the adult are delivered:
   A. 1 every 5 compressions.
   B. 2 every 30 compressions.
   C. 5 per minute.
   D. 15 per minute.

7. If CPR is effective, which of the following will happen?
   A. The patient's skin will turn blue.
   B. The patient's pupils will dilate.
   C. Another rescuer may detect a carotid pulse during compressions.
   D. The other rescuer will find it difficult to ventilate.

8. When providing external chest compressions for the adult patient:
   A. only one hand is used.
   B. the fingers must be kept off the patient's chest.
   C. the hands must point toward the patient's head.
   D. the fingers must be firmly placed between the patient's ribs.

9. CPR can, when necessary, be interrupted for a maximum of _____ seconds.
   A. 5
   B. 7
   C. 9
   D. 10

10. For CPR purposes, a child is considered anyone from _____ to the onset of puberty.
    A. 6 months   C. 2 years
    B. 1 year   D. 8 years

11. When providing CPR, which of the following maneuvers is recommended for use on a child?
    A. head hyperextension   C. jaw-thrust
    B. neutral head position   D. head-tilt, chin-lift

12. The recommended location for assessing a pulse in an infant is the:
    A. apical pulse.   C. radial pulse.
    B. carotid pulse.   D. brachial pulse.

13. The CPR compression site for an infant is located on the midline of the chest:
    A. two finger-widths above the xiphoid process.
    B. one finger-width below the nipples.
    C. one finger-width above the nipples.
    D. three finger-widths below the xiphoid process.

14. During CPR, ventilations for infants and children are delivered at a rate of:
    A. 1 breath every 5 compressions.
    B. 1 breath every 30 compressions.
    C. 2 breaths every 5 compressions.
    D. 2 breaths every 30 compressions.

15. The compression rate for CPR being applied to an infant is at least _____ per minute.
    A. 40   C. 80
    B. 60   D. 100

16. Ineffective CPR will occur if:
    A. the breastbone is compressed.
    B. compression and release times are equal.
    C. the patient is on a hard surface.
    D. proper hand position is not maintained.

17. The majority of patients who are defibrillated are in which heart rhythm?
    A. ventricular fibrillation   C. pulseless electrical activity
    B. ventricular tachycardia   D. asystole

18. The upper chest electrode pad is placed on the:
    A. left side.   C. right side.
    B. midline.   D. suprasternal notch.

19. You have used an automated external defibrillator to deliver a shock to a patient and have been directed to check breathing and pulse. The patient has a pulse but is not breathing. You should:
    A. provide CPR.   C. leave the defibrillator attached.
    B. unhook the defibrillator leads.   D. recharge the defibrillator.

20. After a shock is delivered using a semi-automated AED, the Emergency Medical Responder should:
    A. continue CPR.   C. remain clear of the device.
    B. press the ANALYZE button.   D. push the PRESS TO SHOCK button.

21. The most common operating problem with AEDs has been found to be:

    A. weak batteries.
    B. improperly attached electrode pads.
    C. broken cables.
    D. inaccurate automatic assessment modes.

22. For two-rescuer CPR on an adult, compressions are delivered at a rate of
    _____ compressions per minute.

    A. 40 to 60   C. 80 to 100
    B. 60 to 80   D. approximately 100

Caring for Medical Emergencies

Reading Assignment: First Responder, 8th Edition, pages 245-301

NOTE: As you complete the reading assignment and the tasks assigned in this workbook, remember that Emergency Medical Responder-level care is assessment based. In general, you will be dealing with categories of medical problems. Most specific illnesses in a particular category will receive the same basic care procedures. Examples of categories include chest pain, respiratory difficulties, altered mental status, diabetic emergencies, abdominal pain, allergic reactions, and poisoning. As a care provider, you will probably begin by personalizing this approach. Then, by the end of the course, you will find that your class has developed a standardized system to "sort out" medical emergencies.

KEY TERMS & DEFINITIONS

Define and explain the following terms from Chapter 9. Textbook page references are provided so that you can check your answers.

1. Define the term **cardiac compromise** and list at least three signs and/or symptoms. (p. 251)

    _____

    _____

    _____

2. Define the term **heart attack** and how it might present in a patient. (pp. 251–252)

    _____

    _____

    _____

3. Define the term **congestive heart failure** and how it might present in a patient. (pp. 254–255)

    _____

    _____

    _____

4. Define the term **chronic obstructive pulmonary disease** (COPD) and how it might present in a patient. (pp. 262–263)

    _____

© 2009 by Pearson Education, Inc. *First Responder*, Eighth Edition, Bergeron et al.

5. Define the term **stroke** and how a patient experiencing a stroke might present. (pp. 264–265)

_____

_____

_____

_____

6. Define the term **seizure** and how a patient experiencing a seizure might present. (pp. 267–268)

_____

_____

_____

_____

7. Define the term **diabetes**. Explain the roles of insulin and glucose within the body. (pp. 268–269)

_____

_____

_____

_____

_____

8. Define the term **anaphylactic shock** and list its possible causes. (p. 282)

_____

_____

_____

_____

9. Compare and contrast the terms **hyperthermia** and **hypothermia**. (pp. 282, 286)

_____

_____

_____

_____

10. What does the term **upper** mean in reference to illicit drugs? (p. 294)

_____

_____

11. What does the term **downer** mean in reference to illicit drugs? (p. 294)

_____

_____

EXERCISES

Complete the following exercises. Answers and/or textbook page references are provided at the back of the workbook. Before looking up your answers, think about your responses and discuss them with other students, Emergency Medical Responders, and emergency care providers.

MEDICAL EMERGENCIES

1. What is the difference between a sign and a symptom?

   _____

   _____

2. List SIX common signs of a medical emergency.

   A. _____

   B. _____

   C. _____

   D. _____

   E. _____

   F. _____

3. List SIX common symptoms of a medical emergency.

   A. _____

   B. _____

   C. _____

   D. _____

   E. _____

   F. _____

4. List the FIVE steps in assessing a patient with a general medical complaint.

   A. _____

   B. _____

   C. _____

   D. _____

   E. _____

SPECIFIC MEDICAL EMERGENCIES

5. Explain how a patient might describe the chest discomfort and other pain felt during an episode of suspected cardiac-related chest pain.

   _____

   _____

_____

_____

6. A patient asks you, "Am I having a heart attack?" How would you answer this question?

_____

_____

7. Complete Table 9.1.

Table 9.1 Signs and Symptoms of Heart Attack and Congestive Heart Failure

	SIGNS	SYMPTOMS	EMERGENCY CARE
	(List three in each column)		
HEART ATTACK			
CONGESTIVE HEART FAILURE (CHF)			

8. Adequate breathing is characterized by a normal respiratory rate, which is the number of breaths per minute; depth, which is the _____ _____ _____, and ease, which is _____ _____ the patient is breathing.

9. List FOUR signs or symptoms of inadequate breathing.

A. _____

B. _____

C. _____

D. _____

10. Match the following.

_____ 1. Stroke   A. Main source of energy for the body

_____ 2. Seizure   B. High blood sugar

_____ 3. Glucose   C. Cerebrovascular accident

_____ 4. Hyperglycemia   D. Irregular electrical brain activity

_____ 5. Anaphylactic shock   E. Severe allergic reaction

11. Should you place an object between the teeth of a convulsing patient? Explain why or why not.

_____

_____

POISONINGS, BITES, AND STINGS

12. List the FOUR routes of poisoning and give an example of each type of poisoning.

    A. _____

    B. _____

    C. _____

    D. _____

13. What is a poison control center and when would an Emergency Medical Responder contact one?

    _____

    _____

    _____

    _____

    _____

14. List TWO signs that are good indicators that a patient has inhaled a poison. What evidence of possible sources should you look for during your scene size-up?

    _____

    _____

15. Emergency care for absorbed poisoning includes moving the patient away from the source of the poison and immediately _____ with _____ all the areas of the patient's body that have been exposed to the poison.

16. Complete Table 9.2 by listing the signs of anaphylactic shock.

    Table 9.2 Signs of Anaphylactic Shock

Skin	
Breathing	
Pulse	
Face	
Mental Status	

© 2009 by Pearson Education, Inc. *First Responder*, Eighth Edition, Bergeron et al.

HEAT EMERGENCIES

17. Define the term **core temperature** and discuss its importance to the EMR when assessing a patient.

_____

_____

_____

_____

18. List FIVE signs or symptoms of heat exhaustion.

   A. _____

   B. _____

   C. _____

   D. _____

   E. _____

19. Why is heat stroke considered a life-threatening emergency?

_____

_____

20. When cooling a heat-emergency patient, it is important to fan the patient but be sure not to

_____ the patient.

COLD EMERGENCIES

21. A state of low body temperature, or generalized cold emergency, is also called _____.

22. When caring for a patient who is hypothermic, list TWO steps that you would DO and TWO steps that are considered DON'Ts.

   DOs: A. _____

           B. _____

   DON'Ts: A. _____

           B. _____

23. A localized cold injury is also known as _____. It is due to a significant

   exposure to cold temperature and mainly occurs in the extremities and in the areas of the

   _____, _____, _____,

   _____, _____ and _____.

24. Explain why you should not give fluid containing alcohol or caffeine to a patient with a localized cold injury.

_____

BEHAVIORAL EMERGENCIES

25. List the FOUR main causes of behavioral change.

    A. _____

    B. _____

    C. _____

    D. _____

26. Explain how to use the following steps/factors to better assess potential violence of patients.

    Scene Size-Up _____

    History _____

    Posture _____

    Verbal activity _____

    Physical activity _____

27. List THREE actions you could take to defuse a violent patient.

    A. _____

    B. _____

    C. _____

28. Complete Table 9.3 by listing FIVE types of drugs that may be abused by patients and TWO signs or symptoms of each.

    Table 9.3 Signs or Symptoms of Drug Abuse

TYPES OF DRUG	SIGNS OR SYMPTOMS

© 2009 by Pearson Education, Inc. *First Responder*, Eighth Edition, Bergeron et al.

PERSONAL DEVELOPMENT 1

Consider the fact that Emergency Medical Responder–level care is assessment based. List as many signs and symptoms of a possible medical emergency in the first box. Next, list some specific diseases or conditions that you encounter as an Emergency Medical Responder.

REMEMBER: Each set of signs/symptoms receives its own special care procedures, helping many different patients without ever requiring the rescuer to make a specific diagnosis.

> **Signs and
> Symptoms**

> **Medical Conditions that may be encountered.
> (Example Heart Attack)**

PERSONAL DEVELOPMENT 2

Start a series of exercises using your residence as the center point. Work outward in radius of 1 mile, 5 miles, and 10 miles to detect both typical and unusual potential sites for environmental emergencies. For example, look for any lakes, canals, sports arenas, parks, or other areas where environmental emergencies might occur. Indicate the type of emergency that may be expected and the reasons you used to justify the classification. Next, determine if the emergency is seasonal or has other limitations. Compare your results with fellow students to begin to focus on the environment in your "response area."

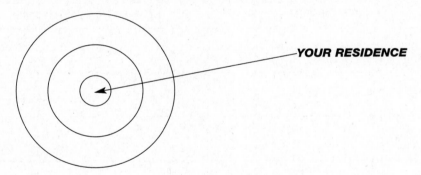

YOUR RESIDENCE

APPLICATION

You are called to the scene of the following patients. Describe your approach and care for each patient by answering the questions that follow each scenario.

1. A 44-year-old man complains of substernal chest pain that developed while playing flag football with his kids. He is alert and oriented; however, he is complaining of mild shortness of breath. Approximately 10 minutes after resting, his pain begins to go away.

    A. Based on these signs and symptoms, what do you think may be wrong with this patient? Why?

    _____

    _____

B. You have no equipment with you and you are the only Emergency Medical Responder on the scene. Describe how you would care for this patient.

_____

_____

2. You are asked to assess an 18-year-old female patient who is upset, crying, and unable to tell you what is wrong with her. A bystander reveals that the patient has broken up with her boyfriend recently and has threatened suicide in the past. The patient is alert and oriented and breathing very rapidly. She complains of difficulty breathing and states that she cannot catch her breath. She also is complaining of tingling to her fingers and lips.

A. Explain how you will approach this patient. What will you say?

_____

_____

B. What might be causing the rapid breathing? How will you care for this patient, and what signs and symptoms will lead you to your choice of an approach for care?

_____

_____

3. A 4-year-old boy was found with some open medicine containers from his mother's purse. He may have taken some iron pills, vitamins, and acetaminophen. He is awake, alert, oriented, and acting "quite normal" according to his mom.

A. How will you determine how best to care for this patient?

_____

_____

B. Think about all of the household items that may become poisons if taken improperly. List a few of those items here and explain how people can best protect themselves and their children from being poisoned.

_____

_____

_____

Discuss these cases with your classmates and compare answers. If you and your classmates disagree on any answers, discuss them with your instructor.

© 2009 by Pearson Education, Inc. *First Responder*, Eighth Edition, Bergeron et al.

ADDITIONAL RESOURCES

You may choose to learn more about this topic. The following references may be helpful:

Hafen, Brent, and Frandsen, *Psychological Emergencies and Crisis Intervention*. Upper Saddle River, NJ: Brady/Prentice Hall.

American Association of Poison Control Centers at http://www.aapcc.org

American Diabetes Association at http://www.diabetes.org

Epilepsy Foundation at http://www.efa.org

Caring for Bleeding, Shock, and Soft-Tissue Injuries

Reading Assignment: First Responder, 8th Edition, pages 302–365

KEY TERMS & DEFINITIONS

Define and explain the following terms from Chapter 10. Textbook page references are provided so that you can check your answers.

1. Define **artery**, **capillary**, and **vein** and explain the function of each. (p. 306)

   _____

   _____

   _____

   _____

   _____

   _____

2. Define the term **perfusion** and list at least three signs of poor perfusion. (p. 307)

   _____

   _____

   _____

   _____

3. What is the difference between a **bandage** and a **dressing?** (p. 317)

   _____

   _____

   _____

4. Define the term **direct pressure** and explain its role in bleeding control. (p. 311)

_____

_____

_____

5. Define **shock** and list some of the common signs and symptoms. (pp. 325, 327)

_____

_____

6. Define the following terms: **superficial burn, partial-thickness burn,** and **full-thickness burn.** (p. 356)

_____

_____

_____

_____

_____

7. Define the **rule of nines.** Explain how it is used to assess burn patients. (pp. 356–357)

_____

_____

_____

_____

_____

EXERCISES

Complete the following exercises. Answers and/or textbook page references are provided at the back of the workbook. Before looking up your answers, think about your responses and discuss them with other students, Emergency Medical Responders, and emergency care providers.

THE BLOOD AND TYPES OF BLEEDING

1. Name the FIVE major functions of the blood.

A. _____

B. _____

C. _____

D. _____

E. _____

2. Give an example of external bleeding and an example of internal bleeding.

External bleeding: _____

Internal bleeding: _____

3. Complete Table 10.1.

Table 10.1 Blood Vessels

Blood Vessel	Function	External Bleeding (Color & Flow)
Artery		
Vein		
Capillary		

4. Of the three types of external bleeding, which is the most serious? Why?

_____

_____

_____

5. Identify the FOUR steps used to control external bleeding shown in Figure 10.1.

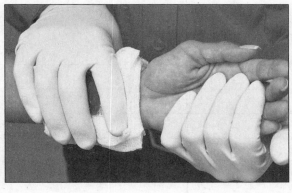

A. _____

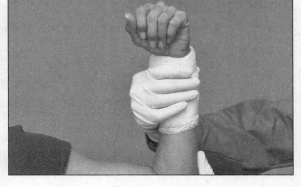

B. _____

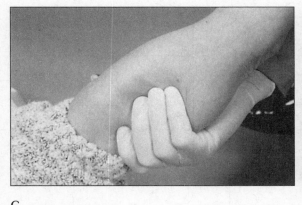

C. _____

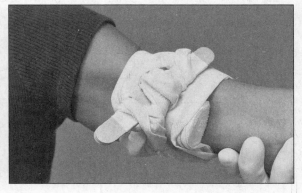

D. _____

Figure 10.1 Controlling External Bleeding.

6. Most cases of external bleeding can best be controlled by applying _____ _____ and _____ .

   The last resort measure is the application of a _____ .

7. For bleeding from an extremity, direct pressure can be used in combination with _____ .

DRESSING AND BANDAGING

8. List FOUR rules that apply to dressing wounds.

   A. _____

   B. _____

   C. _____

   D. _____

9. List FIVE rules that apply to bandaging wounds.

   A. _____

   B. _____

   C. _____

   D. _____

   E. _____

INTERNAL BLEEDING

10. List the common signs and symptoms of internal bleeding.

    _____

    _____

    _____

    _____

11. You may conclude that there is internal bleeding if the patient has the signs and symptoms of

    _____ .

12. List the common signs and symptoms of shock.

    Signs

    _____

    _____

    _____

    _____

Symptoms

_____

_____

_____

_____

13. List the steps that an Emergency Medical Responder should perform when caring for a patient with suspected internal bleeding.

A. _____

B. _____

C. _____

D. _____

E. _____

F. _____

G. _____

H. _____

I. _____

J. _____

NOTE: Emergency Medical Responder protocols in your area may call for the administration of oxygen.

SHOCK

14. Define the term **shock** and list several causes.

_____

_____

_____

15. The body reacts to damage from injury and tries to compensate for that damage. What changes in vital signs might you expect to see for someone with internal bleeding?

_____

_____

_____

16. Describe the signs of shock on a patient.

A. Entire body assessment: _____

B. Mental status: _____

C. Breathing: _____

D. Pulse: _____

E. Skin: _____

© 2009 by Pearson Education, Inc. *First Responder*, Eighth Edition, Bergeron et al.

F. Face: _____

G. Eyes: _____

17. List the symptoms of shock.

_____

_____

_____

_____

_____

18. List at least five things the Emergency Medical Responder can do to care for a patient who is showing the signs and symptoms of shock:

A. _____

B. _____

C. _____

D. _____

E. _____

TYPES OF INJURIES

19. Explain the difference between a closed and an open soft-tissue injury.

_____

_____

20. MATCH the letter of the description (right) to the correct wound (left).

_____ 1. Avulsion   A. Cutting off a finger

_____ 2. Amputation   B. Jagged-edged cut

_____ 3. Bruise   C. Minor open wound

_____ 4. Incision   D. Smooth-edged cut

_____ 5. Laceration   E. Tearing loose of skin

_____ 6. Penetration   F. Both an entrance and exit wound

_____ 7. Perforation   G. Shallow to deep puncture

_____ 8. Scratch   H. Closed wound that causes skin discoloration

21. List the steps in the care of an open wound.

A. _____

B. _____

C. _____

D. _____

E. _____

F. _____

G. _____

22. Although you generally do not remove an impaled object, when and why might you need to remove it?

_____

_____

23. What type of dressing is used on sucking chest wounds? Why?

_____

_____

BURNS

24. List the FIVE major causes of burns and the sources that cause them.

A. _____

B. _____

C. _____

D. _____

E. _____

25. List the areas of the body where partial-thickness burns are considered major burns. Explain why.

_____

_____

_____

26. Use the rule of nines to indicate correct percentages for each area of the body shown in Figure 10.2.

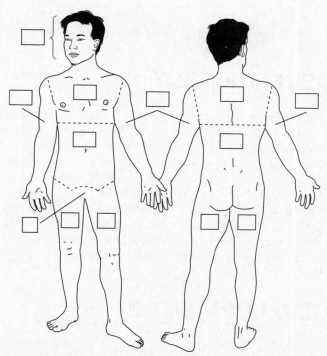

Figure 10.2   The rule of nines.

© 2009 by Pearson Education, Inc. *First Responder*, Eighth Edition, Bergeron et al.

27. Complete the missing steps in caring for thermal burns.

A. Complete a scene size-up before initiating care.

B. Alert dispatch.

C. _____.

D. For minor burns, flush burned area with cool water.

E. For major burns, _____.

F. Prevent further contamination.

G. Cover with dry, sterile dressing.

H. Do not _____.

I. Do not _____.

J. Give special care to the _____.

K. Give special care to the _____.

L. Because burns to the face or exposure to smoke may cause airway problems,

_____.

28. When caring for a patient who is the victim of a chemical burn, you should flush the area with water

for at least _____ minutes.

What is your next step?_____

What would you do if the patient complained that he felt burning again?

_____

_____

_____

PERSONAL DEVELOPMENT 1

Members of the EMS system are often asked to help local groups, organizations, and clubs with member health education. Assume that this will happen to you and that last year an Emergency Medical Responder gave a lecture on basic life support (specifically, CPR). For your topic, select the "GOLDEN HOUR" and the importance of caring for shock. For a start, outline, with terms and definitions, an introduction to the development of shock. Then explain how Emergency Medical Responders can save lives by initiating care that can often prevent shock or limit the rate of its development.

As you continue to learn more about patient assessment and care, continue to develop this talk on shock. How well do you think most persons understand the importance of this subject? Remember, unless people know what Emergency Medical Responders do and how important initial response can be, then public support may be lacking for program growth and development.

PERSONAL DEVELOPMENT 2

Care for soft-tissue injuries often begins before the Emergency Medical Responder arrives at the emergency scene. This is generally the case at sporting events. Some common procedures can hamper assessment and proper care. Having an injured athlete (sprained ankle) walk to "work out the pain" can be a very serious problem. In some instances, the use of ice placed directly on the skin may worsen the patient's condition. What can you and your classmates do to help?

Have your instructor help you organize face-to-face and telephone interviews with local coaches and athletic directors to begin preplanning for emergencies. Take the attitude that you are collecting information on needs rather than investigating procedures that may hamper assessment and care. As you learn from the people who have the need, you can slowly (at first) educate them as to what Emergency Medical Responders hope to find when they arrive and how persons at the scene can help the EMS system provide professional-level care for a properly assessed patient.

APPLICATION

You have been dispatched to an unknown problem at a local oil refinery. Upon arrival you find an approximately 50-year-old male who was injured when a 55-gallon drum of oil was dropped and struck his chest and abdomen. He is alert but confused and has no obvious external injuries. His respirations are 20 and shallow, his pulse is 118 and weak, and his skin is pale and moist. Describe your approach and care for this patient by answering the following questions:

1. What is your first concern for this patient and why?

   _____

   _____

2. How will you determine if he might be bleeding internally?

   _____

   _____

3. What is this man's priority for transport and what will you do for him while awaiting the ambulance?

   _____

   _____

4. The patient becomes unresponsive while you are caring for him. What will your next actions be?

   _____

   _____

Discuss this case with your classmates and compare answers. If you and your classmates disagree on any answers, discuss them with your instructor.

ADDITIONAL RESOURCES

You may choose to learn more about this topic. The following reference may be helpful:

Campbell, John, M.D., *International Trauma Life Support for Prehospital Care Providers*. Upper Saddle River, NJ: Brady/Prentice Hall.

Caring for Muscle and Bone Injuries

Reading Assignment: First Responder, 8th Edition, pages 366–431

KEY TERMS & DEFINITIONS

Define and explain the following terms from Chapter 11. Textbook page references are provided so that you can check your answers.

1. What is the importance of assessing circulation, sensation, and motor function in an injured extremity? (p. 369)

   _____
   _____
   _____

2. Define the term **mechanism of injury**. Why is it important for the Emergency Medical Responder to consider the mechanism of injury? (pp. 372–376)

   _____
   _____
   _____

3. Briefly define each of the following terms. (p. 375)

   fracture _____

   dislocation _____

   sprain _____

   strain _____

4. Define the term **position of function** and its role in splinting. (pp. 390–393)

   _____
   _____
   _____
   _____

© 2009 by Pearson Education, Inc. *First Responder*, Eighth Edition, Bergeron et al.

5. Define the term **concussion** and list TWO associated signs and symptoms. (p. 409)

_____

_____

_____

6. Describe the term **contusion** and list TWO possible causes. (p. 409)

_____

_____

_____

7. What is a **flail chest** and how does it differ from a "simple" rib fracture? (p. 425)

_____

_____

_____

EXERCISES

Complete the following exercises. Answers and/or textbook page references are provided at the back of the workbook. Before looking up your answers, think about your responses and discuss them with other students, Emergency Medical Responders, and emergency care providers.

THE MUSCULOSKELETAL SYSTEM

1. List the FOUR major functions of the musculoskeletal system.

   A. _____

   B. _____

   C. _____

   D. _____

2. List the FOUR structures of the axial skeleton.

   A. _____

   B. _____

   C. _____

   D. _____

3. Label the bones of the appendicular skeleton shown in Figure 11.1.

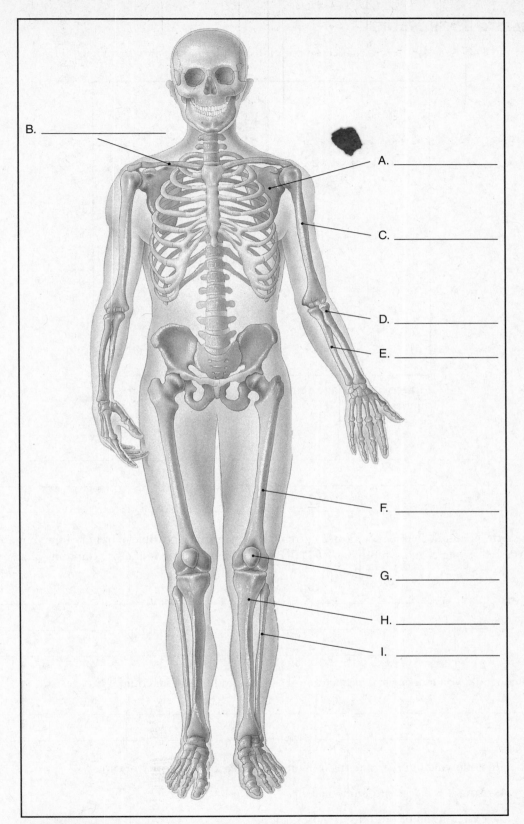

B. _____

A. _____

C. _____

D. _____

E. _____

F. _____

G. _____

H. _____

I. _____

Figure 11.1 Bones of the appendicular skeleton.

INJURIES TO EXTREMITIES

4. List the THREE major forces that cause musculoskeletal injuries shown in Figure 11.2.

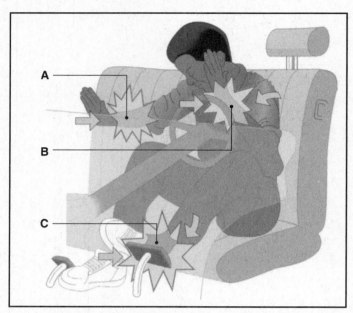

Figure 11.2 Major forces that cause musculoskeletal injuries.

A. _____

B. _____

C. _____

5. The term "painful, swollen, deformed extremity" covers every possible extremity injury. In addition to these three signs and symptoms, list THREE other common signs and/or symptoms of an extremity injury.

A. _____

B. _____

C. _____

6. When would you assess distal circulation, sensation, and motor function? Why?

_____

_____

7. Label the following injuries in terms of high, medium, or low priority of care.

_____ A. Arm, lower leg, and individual ribs

_____ B. Extremity injury (no distal pulse)

_____ C. Rib cage

_____ D. Skull

_____ E. Spine

_____ F. Thigh

_____ G. Pelvis

8. List the SIX steps in caring for an injured extremity.

A. _____

B. _____

C. _____

D. _____

E. _____

F. _____

NOTE: Medical direction may allow you to reposition an injured extremity if there is no distal pulse. Follow local protocols.

SPLINTING

9. Name TWO types of splints: _____ and _____.

Give examples of each.

_____

_____

10. The text lists 14 rules for splinting. Pick four and explain why each is important.

A. _____ _____

B. _____ _____

C. _____ _____

D. _____ _____

11. Match the letter of the splint of choice to the upper extremity injury listed on the left. Answers may be used more than once or not at all.

_____ 1. Upper arm, near shoulder   **A.** Sling and swathe

_____ 2. Hand   **B.** Tie between folded pillows

_____ 3. Elbow   **C.** Wrist sling and swathe

_____ 4. Forearm bone   **D.** Rolled blanket, sling, and swathe

_____ 5. Wrist bones   **E.** Cardboard splint

12. What type of splints would you use for injuries to the following extremities?

Ankle _____

Knee _____

Thigh _____

Hip _____

© 2009 by Pearson Education, Inc. *First Responder*, Eighth Edition, Bergeron et al.

INJURIES TO THE HEAD, SPINE, AND CHEST

13. List as many of the signs and symptoms of a head injury as you can think of before comparing your answers to the text.

14. Complete this list of steps in caring for a patient with a head injury.

    A. Maintain an open airway.
    B. _____.
    C. Keep the patient still.
    D. Control _____.
    E. Talk to the responsive patient.
    F. Dress and bandage _____ wounds and _____ penetrating objects.
    G. Provide care for shock.
    H. _____
    I. Monitor mental status.
    J. Provide emotional support.
    K. Be prepared for _____.
    L. Arrange to transport as soon as possible.

15. Write the names of the sections of the spinal column shown in Figure 11.3.

    A. _____
    B. _____
    C. _____
    D. _____
    E. _____

© 2009 by Pearson Education, Inc. *First Responder*, Eighth Edition, Bergeron et al.

92 **Module 5** Illness and Injury

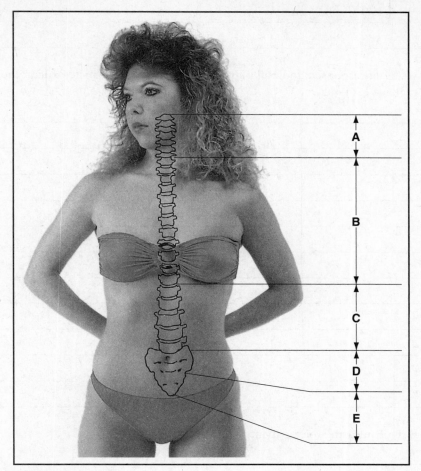
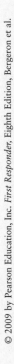

© 2009 by Pearson Education, Inc. *First Responder*, Eighth Edition, Bergeron et al.

Figure 11.3 The spinal column.

16. Indicate which of the following are signs and symptoms of spinal injury (S), flail chest (F), or both (B).

_____ 1) Weakness to arms and legs

_____ 2) Paradoxical movement/deformity

_____ 3) Loss of bowel/bladder control

_____ 4) Guarding

_____ 5) Difficulty breathing

_____ 6) Paralysis to arms or legs

_____ 7) Deformity

17. List SEVEN rules of caring for patients with spinal injuries that are found in the text.

Rule 1: _____

Rule 2: _____

Rule 3: _____

Rule 4: _____

Rule 5: _____

Rule 6: _____

Rule 7: _____

18. Your patient is an unresponsive football player who is wearing a helmet. Explain the steps that you will take to manage his injury.

_____

_____

_____

_____

_____

_____

_____

_____

_____

_____

_____

_____

19. List the FIVE steps in caring for a patient with a flail chest.

A. _____

B. _____

C. _____

D. _____

E. _____

PERSONAL DEVELOPMENT 1

One way to test your understanding of a subject is to try to explain parts of the subject to children. Begin to develop a lesson plan to present to children, perhaps at a local elementary school. Your topic will be the assessment and care of injuries to the bones and joints.

Divide your talk into three parts: (1) How does the fact that bones are alive affect the ways in which they are injured? (2) How do EMS personnel assess the injuries? (3) Why are certain initial care procedures done? Remember, many children have been taught to think of bones as hard, "rocklike" material, not living tissues requiring food and oxygen. Often, children do not relate what they know about tissue healing (e.g., scraped knee) to injured bones.

PERSONAL DEVELOPMENT 2

Arrange through your instructor to interview (face to face or by phone) patients who have received field EMS care for bone injuries. The patients should be those who were responsive throughout their assessment and care. As you talk to these patients, keep track of what they can tell you about what frightened them

© 2009 by Pearson Education, Inc. *First Responder*, Eighth Edition, Bergeron et al.

and what pain was caused by the care. Afterward, decide how you would communicate with such patients to help reduce their fears and to help prepare them for pain during care.

APPLICATION

You have been dispatched to a warehouse for a possible fractured leg. Upon arrival you find an approximately 30-year-old male patient lying on the warehouse floor in obvious distress. A coworker is holding the patient's right leg and explains that the man was struck on his leg by the forks of a fast-moving forklift. Describe your approach and care for this patient by answering the following questions:

1. How will you approach this patient? What will be your priority?

   _____
   _____

2. Once you have determined that his ABCs are okay, how will you go about assessing the extremity?

   _____
   _____
   _____
   _____
   _____

3. What could you use as a splint? (Be creative.)

   _____
   _____

Discuss this case with your classmates and compare answers. If you and your classmates disagree on any answers, discuss them with your instructor.

ADDITIONAL RESOURCES

You may wish to learn more about this topic. The following reference may be helpful.

Campbell, John, M.D., *International Trauma Life Support for Prehospital Care Providers*. Upper Saddle River, NJ: Brady/Prentice Hall.

Caring for the Geriatric Patient

Reading Assignment: First Responder, 8th Edition, pages 432–445

KEY TERMS & DEFINITIONS

Define and explain the following terms from Chapter 12. Textbook page references are provided so that you can check your answers.

1. Define the term **elderly** and explain why we must become more knowledgeable and proficient at caring for this segment of our population. (p. 433)

   _____

   _____

2. Define the term **mobility** and discuss what part the lack of mobility plays in the well-being of the geriatric patient. (p. 435)

   _____

   _____

   _____

3. Define the term **osteoporosis** and describe how this affects the elderly patient. (p. 439)

   _____

   _____

   _____

EXERCISES

Complete the following exercises. Answers and/or textbook page references are provided at the back of the workbook. Before looking up your answers, think about your responses and discuss them with other students, Emergency Medical Responders, and emergency care providers.

© 2009 by Pearson Education, Inc. *First Responder*, Eighth Edition, Bergeron et al.

CHARACTERISTICS OF THE GERIATRIC PATIENT

1. Many elderly patients may have multiple illnesses at any one time. Describe how this might make it difficult for you when providing care.

    _____

    _____

    _____

2. List THREE characteristics common to the geriatric patient and explain how each might affect the care you provide.

    A. _____

    B. _____

    C. _____

AGE-RELATED CHANGES

3. List THREE body systems and describe how the aging process affects them.

    A. _____

    B. _____

    C. _____

4. List THREE things common to the geriatric patient that may make it more difficult for you to complete a quick and efficient assessment.

    A. _____

    B. _____

    C. _____

5. List THREE illnesses common to the geriatric patient.

    A. _____

    B. _____

    C. _____

PERSONAL DEVELOPMENT

Becoming comfortable with the assessment and care of the geriatric population will take time and experience. One way to accelerate the process is to spend more time interacting with older patients. You might want to visit a convalescent home in your area and volunteer to practice taking histories and vital signs on the patients. Many of the residents of these facilities have wonderful stories to tell and would benefit greatly from the interaction you would provide. Before doing so, check with your instructor to make sure it is appropriate and allowed by your training agency or institution. Be sure to take a notepad and paper with you and record as much history as you can. Do not record names because this may be a violation of privacy. Discuss with your classmates your experience and ask them to share theirs as well.

© 2009 by Pearson Education, Inc. *First Responder*, Eighth Edition, Bergeron et al.

APPLICATION

You have been dispatched for a fall victim on the third floor of a senior housing facility. Upon arrival you find an elderly women who is wedged between the toilet and the tub in her bathroom. She is very confused, screams with pain any time you attempt to move her, and is shivering. The best you can tell is that she has been there for approximately 12 hours. Describe your approach to the scene and the care for the patient by answering the following questions:

1. How will you approach this situation? What will be your first priority?

_____

_____

_____

_____

2. What resources might you use to get more of a history?

_____

_____

_____

_____

3. How will you get her moved from the bathroom floor and down the stairs?

_____

_____

_____

_____

Discuss this case with your classmates and compare your answers. If you and your classmates disagree on any answers, discuss them with your instructor.

ADDITIONAL RESOURCES

You may wish to learn more about this topic. The following references may be helpful.

An excellent article on assessment of the geriatric patient can be found at
http://www.aafp.org/afp/20000215/1089.html

http://www.andthoushalthonor.org/ "And Thou Shalt Honor" is a PBS documentary series on the growing elderly population in the United States and how we can best prepare to care for them.

MODULE 5 REVIEW

This self-test has been designed for you to take after you have completed the Reading Assignment, Key Terms & Definitions, and Exercises for Chapters 9, 10, 11, and 12. The answers and page references are given at the end of the workbook.

CIRCLE the letter of the correct answer to each question.

1. A patient is short of breath and complains of pain in his left arm and jaw. You must care for this patient as though he may be experiencing:
   A. congestive heart failure.   C. a heart attack.
   B. a seizure.   D. a stroke.

2. A 65-year-old man complains of a severe headache. His speech is slurred and he has weakness on one side of his body. You suspect this patient may be experiencing:
   A. hyperglycemia.   C. a stroke.
   B. a heart attack.   D. congestive heart failure.

3. A 70-year-old woman with a history of emphysema is complaining of severe fatigue. She is very short of breath, has blue lips and nail beds, and presents with swollen ankles. The patient denies any chest pain. You should suspect:
   A. congestive heart failure.
   B. hyperventilation.
   C. heart attack.
   D. stroke or prelude to altered mental status.

4. A patient with a history of cardiac problems is suffering from an episode of chest pain. He asks you to help him take the medication given to him by his doctor. You should:
   A. call his doctor for directions.
   B. wait for the next level of care to arrive.
   C. help him take the medicine per local protocols.
   D. suggest a double dose because this is an emergency.

5. A patient describing chest pain and showing signs of possible heart attack should be placed:
   A. flat on his back.
   B. on his side.
   C. on his back with legs elevated.
   D. in a comfortable position.

6. The primary responsibility of an Emergency Medical Responder providing care for a patient having a grand mal seizure is to:
   A. place a bite stick in the patient's mouth.
   B. hold the patient still during convulsions.
   C. protect the patient from injury.
   D. protect the patient from embarrassment.

7. A 3-year-old has ingested a poisonous chemical and is unresponsive. You should first:
   A. assure a clear airway.
   B. immediately induce vomiting.
   C. dilute the poison by providing milk or water.
   D. call the poison control center.

© 2009 by Pearson Education, Inc. *First Responder*, Eighth Edition, Bergeron et al.

8. If you are caring for a patient who has been bitten by a venomous snake and transport will be delayed for more than 5 hours, you should:

   A. cut open the wound and let it drain.
   B. pack the site in ice.
   C. apply a constricting band above and below the site.
   D. cut open the bite and suck out the venom.

9. You find a 25-year-old female collapsed and unresponsive on a sports field. Her pupils are dilated, her skin is hot and dry, and her pulse is rapid and strong. These signs indicate possible:

   A. heat stroke.
   B. shock.
   C. diabetic coma.
   D. heat cramps.

10. Which of the following would be an effective water temperature to rewarm a deep local cold injury (frostbitten or frozen part) in cases where transport is delayed?

   A. 70°F
   B. 98.6°F
   C. 104°F
   D. 110°F

11. In late or deep local cold injury (frostbite), the skin often appears:

   A. cherry red.
   B. white and waxy.
   C. deep blue and shining.
   D. light red and dull.

12. The typical adult has about _____ pints of blood.

   A. 6
   B. 8
   C. 12
   D. 14

13. Blood is carried away from the heart to the rest of the body via these vessels.

   A. veins
   B. venules
   C. capillaries
   D. arteries

14. The exchange of nutrients and waste products between the blood and the body's cells takes place at the level of the:

   A. capillaries.
   B. veins.
   C. arteries.
   D. arterioles.

15. Bright red blood spurting from a wound indicates _____ bleeding.

   A. venous
   B. arterial
   C. capillary
   D. venule

16. The best method to control most external bleeding is:

   A. pressure points.
   B. elevation.
   C. a tourniquet.
   D. direct pressure.

17. In most cases of severe internal bleeding, you usually will see the signs and symptoms of:

   A. coma.
   B. shock.
   C. lung shock.
   D. fainting.

18. A patient developing shock is very thirsty. You should give:

   A. nothing by mouth.
   B. cold water.
   C. salty water.
   D. warm liquids.

19. Except for a few special cases, impaled objects should:

    A. not be removed.
    B. be removed if they are loose.
    C. be removed if the impalement is shallow.
    D. be removed to stop bleeding.

20. A responsive patient has a simple nosebleed. You should:

    A. pack the nostrils with cotton and have the patient lean back.
    B. pinch the nostrils shut and have the patient lean back.
    C. pinch the nostrils shut and have the patient lean forward.
    D. allow the bleeding to stop on its own.

21. Your first concern for a patient who has an injury to the mouth is to:

    A. pack the mouth with gauze.
    B. stop all bleeding inside the mouth.
    C. tilt the head forward.
    D. ensure an open airway.

22. A patient is bleeding profusely from a puncture wound to the neck. The blood is bright red, some-times spurting from the wound. You should:

    A. pinch off the ends of the severed vessel, taking care not to close the airway.
    B. apply the carotid artery pressure point technique.
    C. apply a pressure dressing to the wound and secure snugly with roller gauze.
    D. apply direct pressure and an occlusive dressing.

23. A burn that involves all the layers of the skin is commonly referred to as a
    _____ burn.

    A. superficial   C. full-thickness
    B. partial-thickness   D. thermal

24. Minor burns may be:

    A. kept dry and dressed.
    B. flushed in cool water and dressed.
    C. dressed in wet dressing.
    D. dressed after the application of burn ointment.

25. Which of the following chemicals should be brushed from the skin rather than washed away with water?

    A. hydrochloric acid   C. sodium hydroxide
    B. dry lime   D. acetic acid

26. An unknown chemical burn to the eye requires at least _____ minutes of flushing with running water.

    A. 5   C. 15
    B. 10   D. 20

27. Before removing the helmet of an injured motorcycle rider, you should first:

    A. cut the chin strap.
    B. determine if the helmet fits snugly.
    C. pad under the shoulders.
    D. remove the face shield.

28. A patient complains of pain when you apply pressure to both sides of the hips. Your best course of action would be to:

    A. tie his legs together.

    B. elevate his legs.

    C. place the patient on his left side.

    D. elevate the shoulders and head.

29. A patient has a painful and deformed ankle injury. You should:

    A. straighten the foot and apply a pillow splint.

    B. tie his ankles together.

    C. immobilize his foot in the position in which it was found, using a pillow splint.

    D. elevate his entire lower extremity.

30. You can immobilize a fractured finger by:

    A. taping the entire finger.

    B. taping the finger to an adjacent, uninjured finger.

    C. wrapping the finger in dressing.

    D. straightening the finger and applying dressing and tape.

31. A patient has a forearm injury involving the elbow. You can secure a pillow or blanket around the forearm and:

    A. apply a swathe.   C. tape the arm to the chest.

    B. bind the arm with a swathe.   D. apply a sling and swathe.

32. Usually, a rescuer cannot tell if a hip injury is a fracture or a dislocation. In cases of suspected hip injury, the best course of action is to:

    A. tie the legs together.

    B. apply long board splints.

    C. wait for the next level of care to arrive.

    D. tie and elevate the legs.

33. When using a rigid splint on a suspected fractured femur, the longest splint should extend from the _____ to past the foot.

    A. knee   C. hip

    B. buttocks   D. waist

34. When caring for a patient who has been injured while wearing a helmet, you should first:

    A. cut the chin strap and remove the helmet.

    B. remove the shoulder pads.

    C. maintain the airway and stabilize the spine.

    D. place the patient on a spine board.

35. You can suspect possible brain injury if there is head trauma and the pupils of the eyes are:

    A. responsive.   C. constricted.

    B. unequal.   D. pale red.

36. Which of the following is NOT a typical sign or symptom of a skull fracture?

    A. difficulty breathing

    B. unequal pupils

    C. bleeding from the ears

    D. blood and clear fluids in the ears and nose

© 2009 by Pearson Education, Inc. *First Responder*, Eighth Edition, Bergeron et al.

37. If a patient has a head injury, you must suspect _____ injuries.

    A. spinal

    B. nasal

    C. eye

    D. ear

38. If a patient has a head injury, the first step in care is to:

    A. perform a complete patient assessment.

    B. stabilize the neck.

    C. establish and maintain an open airway.

    D. stabilize the entire body.

39. A patient with a head injury has clear fluids draining from the nose. You should:

    A. apply direct pressure with a dressing.

    B. pack the nostrils with dressing.

    C. pack the nostrils and ears with cotton.

    D. not attempt to stop the flow.

40. A patient has an object penetrating the skull. You should:

    A. not remove the object, but stabilize it.

    B. remove the object and apply loose dressings.

    C. do nothing and wait for the next level of care to arrive.

    D. remove the object and apply pressure dressings.

41. A persistent erection of the penis that indicates spinal injury is known as:

    A. incontinence.   C. priapism.

    B. penis erecti.   D. plagiarism.

42. If you must remove a helmet, be sure that:

    A. you have a spine board in position for immobilizing the patient.

    B. your partner is stabilizing the head and maintaining it in-line with the body.

    C. you have called medical direction for permission to remove the helmet.

    D. your partner has called for additional EMS assistance.

43. The Emergency Medical Responder's role in immobilizing a patient with a spinal injury is to:

    A. stabilize the patient's head and neck and transport.

    B. stabilize the patient's head and neck and wait for the next level of care.

    C. immobilize the patient to a backboard and transport.

    D. immobilize the patient to a backboard and wait for the next level of care.

44. Oftentimes a patient with chest injury will hold his hand across the injured side to stabilize it. This is known as guarding, or:

    A. self-protection.   C. detailing.

    B. flailing.   D. self-splinting.

45. The priority when caring for a patient with a fractured rib is:

    A. stabilizing the fracture.

    B. assuring adequate respirations by providing oxygen.

    C. assessing for further injury.

    D. splinting the fracture.

46. Most states have laws that require Emergency Medical Responders to report suspected cases of:
    A. dementia.
    B. abuse and neglect.
    C. Alzheimer's disease.
    D. overdose

47. The aging process can cause a degeneration of the heart's electrical system, which can lead to:
    A. hearing loss.
    B. vision loss.
    C. dysrhythmias.
    D. stroke (brain attack).

48. All of the following are ways the respiratory system is affected by the aging process EXCEPT:
    A. increased strength of respiratory muscles.
    B. decreased flexibility of the chest.
    C. collapse of the smaller airways.
    D. loss of elasticity.

49. The inability to retain urine or feces is called:
    A. dementia.
    B. aphasia.
    C. priapism.
    D. incontinence.

50. Geriatric patients are often less able to defend against illness and may take much longer to recover when they do become ill. This often results in:
    A. multiple simultaneous illnesses.
    B. forgetting doctor appointments.
    C. taking the wrong medications.
    D. hearing loss.

Childbirth

Reading Assignment: First Responder, 8th Edition, pages 447–480

KEY TERMS & DEFINITIONS

Define and explain the following terms from Chapter 13. Textbook page references are provided so that you can check your answers.

1. Define the term **fetus** and explain its average period of development. (p. 451)

   _____

   _____

   _____

2. Define the function of the **uterus** (womb). (p. 451)

   _____

   _____

   _____

3. Explain the term **crowning** and what it indicates about the labor process. (p. 451)

   _____

   _____

   _____

4. Describe the role of the **amniotic sac** during pregnancy. (p. 452)

   _____

   _____

   _____

5. Describe the role of the **placenta** during pregnancy. (p. 452)

   _____

   _____

   _____

6. Explain the purpose of the **umbilical cord** during pregnancy. (p. 452)

_____

_____

_____

7. Explain the difference between **contraction time** and **interval time.** (p. 452)

_____

_____

_____

8. What is meant by **false labor,** or Braxton Hicks contractions? (p. 453)

_____

_____

EXERCISES

Complete the following exercises. Answers and/or textbook page references are provided at the back of the workbook. Before looking up your answers, think about your responses and discuss them with other students, Emergency Medical Responders, and emergency care providers.

UNDERSTANDING CHILDBIRTH

1. Describe the THREE stages of labor and when each begins and ends.

   A. _____   _____

   B. _____   _____

   C. _____   _____

2. Explain how contractions progress during labor.

   _____

   _____

   _____

3. List the indications of an imminent delivery.

   A. _____   _____

   B. _____   _____

   C. _____   _____

4. Name the structures of pregnancy in Figure 13.1.

   A. _____   _____

   B. _____   _____

   C. _____   _____

D. _____

E. _____

F. _____

G. _____

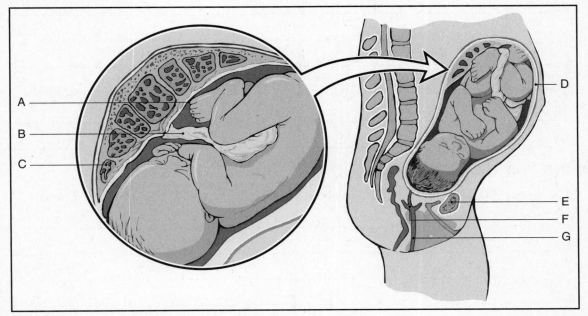

Figure 13.1 The structures of pregnancy.

DELIVERY

5. List EIGHT questions that you must ask the mother as you begin to evaluate her to see if delivery is imminent.

A. _____

B. _____

C. _____

D. _____

E. _____

F. _____

G. _____

H. _____

6. List the SIX steps in preparing for an imminent delivery.

A. _____

B. _____

C. _____

D. _____

© 2009 by Pearson Education, Inc. *First Responder*, Eighth Edition, Bergeron et al.

E. _____

F. _____

7. List FOUR items that should be worn as personal protective equipment during a prehospital delivery.

A. _____

B. _____

C. _____

D. _____

8. When the baby's head appears, which is known as _____, how should you position your hands?

_____

_____

CARING FOR THE NEWBORN

9. List the first SIX steps in caring for a newborn.

A. _____

B. _____

C. _____

D. _____

E. _____

F. _____

10. If the baby does not breathe on his own by the time you clear the airway, what should you do to encourage him to breathe?

_____

_____

_____

_____

_____

_____

11. Complete Table 13.1.

CARING FOR THE MOTHER

12. Describe how to collect and save the placenta and explain why it should be saved.

_____

_____

_____

_____

_____

© 2009 by Pearson Education, Inc. *First Responder*, Eighth Edition, Bergeron et al.

Table 13.1 Caring for a Newborn

IF THERE IS A PULSE, BUT YOU SEE THIS . . .	YOU SHOULD DO THIS
Breathing rate is inadequate.	
Heart rate is at least 100 beats per minute and spontaneous breathing is present.	
Heart rate less than 60 beats per minute.	

13. Explain the steps for controlling vaginal bleeding in the mother following a delivery.

_____

_____

_____

_____

_____

_____

_____

_____

_____

_____

_____

_____

_____

_____

COMPLICATIONS AND EMERGENCIES

14. Match each condition or complication with the definition.

_____ 1) Meconium staining   A. Fetus delivers before it can survive on its own

_____ 2) Miscarriage   B. Infant's fecal material mixes with amniotic fluid

_____ 3) Stillborn birth   C. Buttocks or both feet deliver first

_____ 4) Breech birth   D. Umbilical cord protrudes from vagina

_____ 5) Prolapsed cord   E. Baby born dead or dies shortly after birth

15. List the SIX steps in caring for a woman who is having a suspected spontaneous abortion.

A. _____

B. _____

C. _____

D. _____

E. _____

F. _____

16. Complete Table 13.2.

Table 13.2 Abnormal Deliveries

IF YOU ENCOUNTER THIS SITUATION . . .	YOU SHOULD . . .
Breech birth	
Prolapsed cord	
Premature birth	

17. A woman who is 8 months pregnant stumbled and fell down several steps landing on her abdomen. Explain your concerns and discuss your care for this patient.

_____

_____

_____

_____

_____

18. A woman who is pregnant has been robbed, beaten, and sexually assaulted. Explain your role in this patient's care.

_____

_____

_____

_____

_____

_____

_____

_____

PERSONAL DEVELOPMENT

Consider and list the things that you believe an Emergency Medical Responder may do for a mother during labor and after a normal delivery to help her emotionally.

_____

_____

_____

_____

_____

_____

_____

_____

Compare your answers with your fellow students. What did you leave out? What factors affected your answers?

_____

_____

_____

© 2009 by Pearson Education, Inc. *First Responder*, Eighth Edition, Bergeron et al.

APPLICATION

You are camping with your family when you are awakened in the middle of the night by a woman scream-ing. You peek out of your tent to see what is the matter and hear a man yelling for help, stating that his wife is in labor. You grab your first-aid kit and head over to the campsite where the woman is located. Upon arrival you find an approximately 25-year-old in moderate to severe distress. She appears to be in the late stages of pregnancy and you are told that the baby is not due for another 2 weeks. Describe your approach and care for this patient by answering the following questions.

1. What is your first priority in approaching this patient?

    _____

    _____

2. What equipment or supplies will you use in assisting this patient?

_____

_____

3. The patient asks to use the bathroom. What should you say and why?

_____

_____

Discuss this case with your classmates and compare your answers. If you and your classmates disagree on any answers, discuss them with your instructor.

ADDITIONAL RESOURCES

You may choose to learn more about this topic. The following reference may be helpful:

Neonatal Resuscitation Program. Dallas, TX: American Heart Association.

Caring for Infants and Children

Reading Assignment: First Responder, 8th Edition, pages 481–526

KEY TERMS & DEFINITIONS

Define and explain the following terms from Chapter 14. Textbook page references are provided so that you can check your answers.

1. Define **soft spot** (fontanelle). Explain the potential causes of a bulging fontanelle and a sunken fontanelle. (p. 492)

   _____

   _____

   _____

2. Explain why children are more likely than adults to become **hypothermic.** (p. 494)

   _____

   _____

   _____

3. What is **blow-by oxygen** and how is it performed as an emergency care procedure? (p. 497)

   _____

   _____

   _____

4. Define the term **dehydration** and explain why children are also easily susceptible to this condition. (p. 508)

   _____

   _____

   _____

5. Explain why **hyperextension** of an infant's neck may be harmful during resuscitation. (p. 496)

   _____

   _____

   _____

6. Explain how to place a small child's or infant's head in a **neutral position** while managing the airway. (p. 497)

_____

_____

_____

7. Define the term **SIDS** and list three signs of this condition. (p. 506)

_____

_____

A. _____

B. _____

C. _____

8. Define the term **near-drowning.** (p. 509)

_____

_____

_____

9. Define the term **neglect** and list three signs of neglect. (p. 520)

_____

_____

_____

10. Define the term **asthma** and describe how it presents in children. (p. 502)

_____

_____

_____

EXERCISES

Complete the following exercises. Answers and/or textbook page references are provided at the back of the workbook. Before looking up your answers, think about your responses and discuss them with other students, Emergency Medical Responders, and emergency care providers.

AGE, SIZE, AND RESPONSE

1. Complete Table 14.1.

© 2009 by Pearson Education, Inc. *First Responder*, Eighth Edition, Bergeron et al.

Table 14.1 Child Classification by Age

CLASSIFICATION	AGE RANGE
Newborn	
Toddler	
	3 to 5 years old
School Age	
	12 to 18 years old

SPECIAL CONSIDERATIONS

2. A child's head is proportionally _____ and _____ relative to his body.

3. On Figure 14.1, label the special considerations you need to take into account when assessing a child.

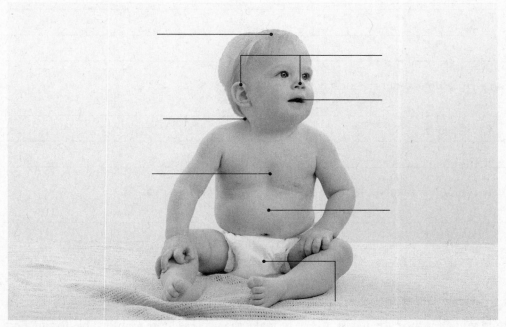

Figure 14.1 Special assessment considerations.

4. Explain why you should never perform blind finger sweeps when trying to clear a foreign body airway obstruction from a child or infant.

_____

_____

_____

© 2009 by Pearson Education, Inc. *First Responder*, Eighth Edition, Bergeron et al.

5. The normal respiratory rate of a(n):

adolescent is from _____ to _____ breaths per minute.

child is from _____ to _____ breaths per minute.

infant is from _____ to _____ breaths per minute.

neonate is from _____ to _____ breaths per minute.

6. Capillary refill should be _____ seconds in the child.

7. If a child patient is NOT breathing, provide artificial ventilations at the rate of 1 breath every _____ to _____ seconds.

PATIENT ASSESSMENT

8. While forming a general impression of a child, list FOUR pieces of critical information you can tell about a child or his condition by simply looking.

   A. _____

   B. _____

   C. _____

   D. _____

9. What can we presume about the airway of a crying child?

   _____

   _____

   _____

10. List FOUR conditions that would indicate a high-priority pediatric patient.

    A. _____

    B. _____

    C. _____

    D. _____

11. How could you alter the patient assessment to make the process more comfortable for an alert but frightened child?

    _____

    _____

    _____

    _____

MANAGING SPECIFIC MEDICAL AND TRAUMA SITUATIONS

12. List FIVE signs of respiratory difficulty (distress) that may indicate a high priority for transport.

    A. _____

    B. _____

C. _____

D. _____

E. _____

13. List eight signs and symptoms of asthma in the pediatric patient.

A. _____

B. _____

C. _____

D. _____

E. _____

F. _____

G. _____

H. _____

14. List THREE causes of seizures in a child.

A. _____

B. _____

C. _____

15. Explain how you would care for a child following a suspected seizure.

_____

_____

_____

_____

16. List THREE medical or trauma emergencies that may cause altered mental status.

A. _____

B. _____

C. _____

17. Shock is also known as _____. How does a child differ from an adult in terms of his ability to compensate for poor perfusion?

_____

18. You may have to provide emotional support to the parents of a SIDS victim. What might you say to comfort the parents?

_____

_____

_____

© 2009 by Pearson Education, Inc. *First Responder*, Eighth Edition, Bergeron et al.

19. Children can usually tolerate fevers well, but be alert for certain signs and symptoms that indicate a serious medical problem. What indications would you look for?

_____

_____

_____

20. Explain why an Emergency Medical Responder may have more success performing a toe-to-head assessment on a small child.

_____

_____

21. A child may suffer rapid heat loss through the top of the _____. Why?

_____

_____

22. List THREE "DOs" when caring for a child who has a fever.

A. _____

B. _____

C. _____

23. List TWO "DON'Ts" when caring for a child who has a fever.

A. _____

B. _____

24. What are the FOUR types of child abuse/neglect you may encounter?

A. _____

B. _____

C. _____

D. _____

25. What is your obligation if you suspect any type of child abuse or neglect?

_____

_____

_____

PERSONAL DEVELOPMENT

Consider how you might feel if you were a parent who had just lost a child to a medical or trauma emergency. Or, what if your child were injured and required emergency transport to the hospital? What would you like the Emergency Medical Responder to do or say to provide emotional support to you?

Compare your answers with your fellow students. What did you leave out? What factors affected your answers?

_____

_____

_____

_____

_____

_____

APPLICATION

You are dispatched to the residence of a child who is not breathing. Upon arrival you find an upset woman clutching what appears to be an approximately 2-year-old girl. Both woman and child are crying. The mother states that the child just stopped breathing and she didn't know what to do. You ask to take a look at the child and discover several bruises that are consistent with abuse. Describe your approach and care for this patient by answering the following questions:

A. How will you approach the patient?

_____

_____

B. What are some typical signs of abuse that you may find when examining children?

_____

_____

C. Should you ask the mother to wait in the other room? Why or why not?

_____

_____

Discuss this case with your classmates and compare your answers. If you and your classmates disagree on any answers, discuss them with your instructor.

ADDITIONAL RESOURCES

You may choose to learn more about this topic. The following references may be helpful:

Eichelberger, Martin R., et al., *Pediatric Emergencies*, 2nd. Ed. Upper Saddle River, NJ: Brady/Prentice Hall.

American SIDS Institute at http://www.sids.org

National Clearinghouse for Child Abuse and Neglect Information at http://nccanch.acf.hhs.gov/index.cfm

Emergency Medical Services for Children at http://www.ems-c.org/

© 2009 by Pearson Education, Inc. *First Responder*, Eighth Edition, Bergeron et al.

MODULE 6 REVIEW

This self-test has been designed for you to take after you have completed the Reading Assignment, Key Terms & Definitions, and Exercises for Chapters 13 and 14. The answers and page references are given at the end of the workbook.

CIRCLE the letter of the correct answer to each question.

1. The developing unborn baby is called a:
   A. placenta.
   B. foramen.
   C. womb.
   D. fetus.

2. The fetus grows and develops inside a protective muscular organ known as the:
   A. umbilical cord.
   B. placenta.
   C. uterus.
   D. cervix.

3. The organ that allows for exchange between the mother's circulatory system and that of the developing unborn baby is the:
   A. amniotic sac.
   B. placenta.
   C. cervix.
   D. foramen.

4. The first stage of labor begins with:
   A. dilation of the cervix.
   B. vaginal contractions.
   C. contractions of the uterus.
   D. placental contractions.

5. The second stage of labor ends with:
   A. full dilation of the cervix.
   B. delivery of the baby.
   C. delivery of the afterbirth.
   D. the start of contractions.

6. The third stage of labor ends with:
   A. full dilation of the cervix.
   B. the start of contractions.
   C. delivery of the placenta.
   D. delivery of the baby.

7. If a woman is having her first baby, labor will usually last approximately _____ hours.
   A. 2   B. 5   C. 16   D. 24

8. Making a final decision about delivery at the scene or arranging transport requires you to:
   A. time the mother's contractions.
   B. feel the abdomen for movement.
   C. check for bleeding from the birth canal.
   D. look to see if any part of the baby is visible.

9. If the amniotic sac does not rupture prior to delivery, you should:
   A. do nothing; it will break once delivery of the baby takes place.
   B. wait until after the delivery and snip it with sterile scissors.
   C. puncture it with your finger and remove the membrane from around the baby's mouth and nose.
   D. transport the mother immediately.

10. In a normal delivery with the mother placed on her back, the baby will be born with face turned

    A. up.
    B. to the right.
    C. down.
    D. to the left.

11. If difficulties arise during the delivery of the baby's upper shoulder, you can assist by gently:

    A. pulling at the baby's shoulders.
    B. guiding the baby's head downward.
    C. guiding the baby's head upward.
    D. gliding your gloved hand into the birth canal.

12. Immediately after the baby is delivered, you should:

    A. clamp or tie the cord.
    B. clear the baby's mouth and nose.
    C. lay the baby on his back.
    D. lift the baby by the feet and slap his buttocks.

13. The baby should begin breathing on his own within _____ of delivery.

    A. 30 seconds
    B. 1 minute
    C. 2 minutes
    D. 4 minutes

14. If the baby does not begin to breathe and his mouth and nose are clear, you should:

    A. begin mouth-to-mask resuscitation.
    B. slap the baby's buttocks.
    C. hold the baby and rub his back or snap a finger on the sole of his foot.
    D. call for immediate transport.

15. When clamping the baby's umbilical cord, the first clamp is placed approximately _____ inches from the baby.

    A. 2
    B. 5
    C. 10
    D. 12

16. The placenta must be:

    A. saved and transported.
    B. allowed to remain in the uterus.
    C. expelled during the baby's delivery.
    D. delivered within 5 minutes of the baby.

17. The first step to control vaginal bleeding after delivery is to:

    A. apply a pressure dressing shaped like a diaper.
    B. place a sanitary pad over the vaginal opening.
    C. massage the uterus.
    D. pack the birth canal with sterile gauze.

18. The part of the baby usually born first in a breech delivery is:

    A. both arms.
    B. the buttocks.
    C. the leg.
    D. the kness.

19. The major role of the Emergency Medical Responder during a breech birth is to:

    A. create and maintain an airway for the baby.
    B. push on the mother's abdomen to increase the strength of contractions.
    C. support the baby's head while it is in the birth canal.
    D. alert the EMS system.

20. A baby is considered premature if it is born prior to the _____ month of pregnancy.
   A. 7th   B. 8th   C. 9th   D. 10th

21. When performing a physical exam of a child, you should:
   A. explain the examination and conduct it at the same rate you would for an adult.
   B. explain the examination and conduct it at a relaxed pace.
   C. explain a step, do the procedure, then explain the next step.
   D. do the examination, explaining each step while you are doing it.

22. The term "toddler" applies to a patient who is from _____ year(s) old.
   A. birth to 1.   C. 2 to 4.
   B. 1 to 3.   D. 3 to 6.

23. A child's body size will "catch up" with his head size by age:
   A. 1   B. 2   C. 3   D. 6

24. Compared to an adult's airway, the child's airway is:
   A. more curved.   C. narrower.
   B. wider.   D. stronger.

25. The child is more prone to hypothermia due to his:
   A. large blood volume.   C. small blood volume.
   B. small skin surface area.   D. large skin surface area.

26. Great care must be taken when employing the head-tilt, chin-lift maneuver on a small child because the procedure may close off the airway due to:
   A. hyperextension.   C. hyperflexion.
   B. hypoextension.   D. hypoflexion.

27. If a child who is developing shock refuses to let you place an oxygen mask on his or her face, you should:
   A. withhold oxygen to avoid conflict.
   B. try to use the blow-by method.
   C. place the mask and insist that the child listen.
   D. stop to explain and quietly place the mask.

28. The purpose of the initial assessment of an infant or a child patient is to detect and care for life-threatening problems associated with:
   A. the ABCs, including development of shock.
   B. breathing and heartbeat.
   C. the ABCs.
   D. airway, breathing, and heartbeat.

29. For a small child who is ill or injured, it is recommended to perform a patient assessment in the following manner:
   A. head-to-toe.   C. front-to-back.
   B. toe-to-head.   D. back-to-front.

30. A respiratory infection that causes tissues in the child's upper airway to become swollen and results in a barking cough, or stridor, is called:

   A. epiglottitis.
   B. cyanosis.
   C. SIDS.
   D. croup.

31. A child is wheezing and is having difficulty exhaling. There are no visible objects in the airway. You should:

   A. give sips of water or provide chipped ice.
   B. avoid placing anything into the child's mouth.
   C. place the child in a supine position.
   D. do not administer oxygen or allow others to do so.

32. Any child who has had a first seizure should:

   A. receive medication.
   B. have a medical evaluation.
   C. be positioned on his or her back.
   D. be questioned about the cause.

33. When a sick child goes into the decompensated shock stage:

   A. there is little that can be done.
   B. he or she will begin to slowly show signs and symptoms of shock.
   C. the signs and symptoms of shock develop rapidly.
   D. the body begins to compensate for low blood sugar.

34. Sudden infant death syndrome is the result of:

   A. unknown factors.
   B. child neglect.
   C. untreated upper respiratory infections.
   D. pneumonia.

35. A child with a high relative skin temperature who is shivering should be:

   A. immersed in cold water.
   B. cooled with rubbing alcohol applied to his or her skin.
   C. undressed down to underwear or diaper and covered with a light blanket.
   D. left fully clothed and covered with a standard blanket should chills develop.

36. Infants are more susceptible to dehydration than are adults because they:

   A. generally vomit more often.
   B. have such small circulating blood volume.
   C. are likely to have less fluid intake.
   D. have much larger heads in proportion to their bodies.

37. A responsive, uninjured toddler who is not nauseous but has the signs of dehydration should be given:

   A. eight ounces of water as soon as possible.
   B. nothing by mouth.
   C. warm liquids to drink.
   D. blowby oxygen.

© 2009 by Pearson Education, Inc. *First Responder*, Eighth Edition, Bergeron et al.

38. When assessing and providing emergency care for a severely injured infant, always begin by:

A. assessing the airway.
B. controlling obvious serious bleeding.
C. immobilizing the spine.
D. covering the child to prevent rapid heat loss.

39. An injured child is found in a child safety seat. Unless rapid removal is required, the best method of removing the child for transport is to:

A. simply remove both the child and seat as a unit.
B. stabilize the child's head and neck and simply remove the child.
C. stabilize the child's head and neck while the child is still secured to the seat and remove the child onto a small rigid board.
D. carefully remove the child, provide care for shock, and wait for the next level of care to arrive to stabilize the head and spine.

40. You suspect a child patient has been abused; however, there are no signs of obvious injury. You should

A. realize that child abuse is a limited problem and that you will probably see few cases.
B. arrange for transport and report your suspicions to the proper authorities.
C. confront the child with a direct question about abuse.
D. keep asking questions, coming back to those about possible previous injuries.

EMS Operations

Reading Assignment: First Responder, 8th Edition, pages 527–552

KEY TERMS & DEFINITIONS

Define and explain the following terms from Chapter 15. Textbook page references are provided so that you can check your answers.

1. Explain the difference between **simple** and **complex** access and the Emergency Medical Responder's role with each. (p. 537)

   _____

   _____

2. Discuss what **CHEMTREC** is and its role in scene safety. (p. 547)

   _____

   _____

   _____

3. Discuss the Emergency Medical Responder's role at a scene where there may be downed power lines. (pp. 545–547)

   _____

   _____

   _____

EXERCISES

Complete the following exercises. Answers and/or textbook page references are provided at the back of the workbook. Before looking up your answers, think about your responses and discuss them with other students, Emergency Medical Responders, and emergency care providers.

© 2009 by Pearson Education, Inc. *First Responder,* Eighth Edition, Bergeron et al.

SAFETY

1. Your first consideration at any emergency scene is your own safety. List steps you should take to assure your own safety.

   _____

   _____

   _____

2. List FOUR steps you should take to minimize your risk at an emergency scene.

   A. _____

   B. _____

   C. _____

   D. _____

MOTOR VEHICLE COLLISIONS

3. Describe in detail the SIX phases of an emergency call:

   A. _____

   B. _____

   C. _____

   D. _____

   E. _____

   F. _____

4. List hazards that Emergency Medical Responders may expect to find at the scene of a vehicle collision.

   _____

   _____

   _____

   _____

5. Complete the following list of the FOUR ways to gain access to patients in a vehicle.

   A. Open the doors.

   B. Enter through _____.

   C. Pry open the _____.

   D. Cut through _____.

6. You find a vehicle on its side and have some simple equipment. List the FOUR precautions you should take to stabilize it.

   A. _____

   B. _____

   C. _____

   D. _____

7. List THREE methods that an Emergency Medical Responder may use to free an occupant caught in the wreckage of a vehicle.

A. _____

B. _____

C. _____

BUILDINGS

8. Is it part of the Emergency Medical Responder's responsibility to know how to open or destroy locks on buildings or have all the tools necessary to do so? _____ Explain.

_____

_____

_____

9. List the FOUR steps in breaking a window to gain entry into a building.

A. _____

B. _____

C. _____

D. _____

HAZARDS

10. List the EIGHT rules an Emergency Medical Responder with little or no training in fighting fires should follow when facing smoke or flames.

A. _____

B. _____

C. _____

D. _____

E. _____

F. _____

G. _____

H. _____

11. Explain what to do if you notice a natural gas leak at an emergency scene.

_____

_____

_____

12. Consider all downed wires to be live. If downed wires are resting on or near a vehicle, what instructions should Emergency Medical Responders give to the vehicle's occupants?

_____

_____

_____

© 2009 by Pearson Education, Inc. *First Responder,* Eighth Edition, Bergeron et al.

13. List the THREE steps to take in a hazardous materials situation. First, _____;
    then set up a _____ and a _____.

14. A HOT zone is the _____ zone, and a COLD zone is the
    _____ zone.

15. List EIGHT items of essential information that should be relayed to the dispatcher regarding a hazardous materials incident.

    A. _____

    B. _____

    C. _____

    D. _____

    E. _____

    F. _____

    G. _____

    H. _____

16. Stay clear of accidents involving radioactive materials. Explain the difference between contamination and exposure.

    _____

    _____

PERSONAL DEVELOPMENT

Create potential scenarios or situations that would benefit you and other rescuers at your level of ability for each of the five situations listed here. Prepare brief outlines of what you personally would need to do to handle each situation. Then practice these procedures as a group.
• Control the scene of a traffic collision.
• Gain access into a typical locked automobile that is in an upright position after a collision.
• Gain access into a typical locked automobile that is resting on its side after a collision.
• Enter a typical family dwelling during a response to a reported medical emergency.
• Safely report details of a hazardous materials incident.

APPLICATION

You have been dispatched to a vehicle collision on an elevated portion of the freeway. Upon arrival you see at least three passenger cars involved and a large tractor trailer rig that has fallen on its side, with the cab section hanging precariously over the side of the freeway. Describe your approach to the scene and the care for the patients by answering the following questions:

1. How will you approach this situation? What will be your priority?

    _____

    _____

    _____

    _____

2. Based on what you know so far, what resources will you request from dispatch?

_____

_____

_____

_____

3. What do you see as your top three hazards at this scene, and how will you manage them?

_____

_____

_____

_____

Discuss this case with your classmates and compare your answers. If you and your classmates disagree on any answers, discuss them with your instructor.

ADDITIONAL RESOURCES

You may choose to learn more about this topic. The following reference may be helpful:

Emergency Response Guidebook 2008. U.S. Department of Transportation.

Multiple-Casualty Incidents, Triage, and the Incident Management System

© 2009 by Pearson Education, Inc. *First Responder*, Eighth Edition, Bergeron et al.

Reading Assignment: First Responder 8th Edition, pages 553–567

KEY TERMS & DEFINITIONS

Define and explain the following terms from Chapter 16. Textbook page references are provided so that you can check your answers.

1. Define the term **multiple-casualty incident** (MCI). (p. 554)

   _____

   _____

   _____

   _____

2. Discuss the role of the Emergency Medical Responder at the scene of an MCI. (p. 555)

   _____

   _____

   _____

   _____

   _____

3. Define the term **Incident Management System** and discuss its role at the scene of an MCI. (p. 555)

   _____

   _____

   _____

_____

_____

4. Define the term **triage.** (p. 556)

_____

_____

5. Explain what each letter in the **START** triage system stands for. (p. 558)

   S _____

   T _____

   A _____

   R _____

   T _____

6. Explain the process of triage and its purpose on the scene of multicasualty incidents. (p. 556)

   _____

   _____

   _____

   _____

   _____

EXERCISES

Complete the following exercises. Answers and/or textbook page references are provided at the back of the workbook. Before looking up your answers, think about your responses and discuss them with other students, Emergency Medical Responders, and emergency care providers.

1. For each of the four triage categories below, describe a patient that might fit into the category:

   A. Immediate _____

   B. Delayed _____

   C. Minor _____

   D. Deceased _____

2. List and discuss the three assessment criteria used in the START triage system.

   A. _____

   B. _____

   C. _____

3. Using the START triage system, categorize each of the following patients who have been involved in a bus rollover incident and discuss your rationale:

© 2009 by Pearson Education, Inc. *First Responder*, Eighth Edition, Bergeron et al.

A. 44-year-old female who is found lying on the ground. She is responsive and complaining of abdominal pain. Respirations are 22 and capillary refill is less than 2 seconds.

_____

_____

B. 20-year-old male with an open and bleeding neck injury. Respirations are 32 and capillary refill time is less than 2 seconds.

_____

_____

C. 30-year-old male who is unresponsive. Respirations are absent and capillary refill is greater than 2 seconds.

_____

_____

D. 15-year-old male who is standing at the scene. He has obvious deformity to his right arm and is in a lot of pain. Respirations are 24 and capillary refill is less than 2 seconds.

_____

_____

E. 60-year-old female lying unresponsive on the ground. No obvious injuries. Respirations are 14 and capillary refill is greater than 2 seconds.

_____

_____

F. 30-year-old male who is responsive and complaining that he cannot move his legs. Respirations are 28 and capillary refill time is 4 seconds.

_____

_____

© 2009 by Pearson Education, Inc. *First Responder*, Eighth Edition, Bergeron et al.

PERSONAL DEVELOPMENT

Triage can be a very difficult concept to implement when you consider that the majority of your training as an Emergency Medical Responder has been focused on identifying and treating life-threatening problems. What happens in many cases is the Emergency Medical Responder successfully triages three or four patients who are relatively stable then comes upon someone who is not breathing. His instinct tells him to stop and provide the indicated care. This stops the triage process in its tracks and is not the best thing for all patients. Discuss with an experienced EMS professional who may have had the duty of triage at the scene of an MCI. Ask them if it was difficult to triage patients without treating them. Ask them to share with you how they overcame the desire to stop and care for critical patients.

ADDITIONAL RESOURCES

You may choose to learn more about this topic. The following references may be helpful:

The START Triage home page: http://www.start-triage.com/

Online training using the START Triage system: http://www.citmt.org/start/

MODULE 7 REVIEW

This self-test has been designed for you to take after you have completed the Reading Assignment, Key Terms & Definitions, and Exercises for Chapters 15 and 16. The answers and page references are given at the end of the workbook.

CIRCLE the letter of the correct answer to each question.

1. Tasks such as evaluating the scene, making the scene safe, and providing care at a motor vehicle collision are:

    A. performed after the ambulance arrives.
    B. performed by police officers before Emergency Medical Responders arrive.
    C. duties of EMS officers.
    D. duties of Emergency Medical Responders.

2. At a motor vehicle collision, you should park your vehicle at least _____ feet from the involved vehicles.

    A. 25   C. 75
    B. 50   D. 100

3. A motor vehicle collision has occurred on a highway, just beyond a curve. The farthest warning device from the scene should be placed at least _____ feet from the involved vehicles.

    A. 250   C. 300
    B. 275   D. 325

4. The simplest way to stabilize an upright vehicle that has come to rest on an inclined road surface is to:

    A. tie a line from the frame to stable objects.
    B. chock the wheels.
    C. chain the vehicle to your own vehicle.
    D. jack one wheel about 2 inches off the ground.

5. Which of the following is the recommended order of access routes to a patient in a motor vehicle?

    A. windows, doors, roof   C. doors, windows, body
    B. doors, windows, trunk   D. roof, trunk, doors

6. The best method of breaking glass in a vehicle door window requires:

    A. striking the glass with a blunt object.
    B. using a blunt tool and hammer.
    C. striking the glass with a sharp object.
    D. using a spring loaded center punch.

7. Before trying to free a patient's arm that is caught in a broken window, you should:

    A. protect the arm with dressing or towels.
    B. fully remove the windshield.
    C. begin by removing the glass that is closest to the arm.
    D. begin by folding away the laminated glass that is closest to the arm.

8. Before cutting a seat belt to free a trapped patient, you should:

    A. move the seat forward.
    B. move the seat backward.

© 2009 by Pearson Education, Inc. *First Responder*, Eighth Edition, Bergeron et al.

C. properly support the patient before tension is released.

D. loosen the anchor bolts of the belt.

9. You find yourself in a smoke-filled room. You should:

A. open a window and clear the smoke.

B. leave, if possible, staying close to the floor.

C. walk from the room using an article of clothing to form a tent over your head.

D. leave by the elevator if possible.

10. A patient is in a stable car that is touching a downed electrical line. There is no fire. The patient should be told to:

A. stay in the car.

B. open the door and jump clear of the car.

C. leave the car by way of a window.

D. calmly open the door and carefully walk away.

11. Once a patient has been triaged, which of the following injuries would be the highest priority?

A. injuries to the spine

B. unresponsive patients with head injuries

C. open chest wounds

D. multiple fractures

12. Under the procedure of triage, severe burns are _____ priority.

A. highest

B. primary

C. lowest

D. secondary

13. At a large disaster scene, injuries that include severe burns, shock, and severe or uncontrolled bleeding are considered:

A. serious but not life threatening.

B. injuries that can wait for care.

C. treatable but life threatening.

D. fatal injuries.

14. A responsive patient with no head or spinal injures has a rapid pulse. Respirations are rapid and shallow. The skin is pale, hot, and dry. Further examination reveals that the pupils are dilated and unresponsive to light. The patient is not paralyzed and has sensation in his extremities. During triage, you must consider this patient to be suffering from:

A. a stroke.

B. shock.

C. heat stroke.

D. hyperglycemia.

15. The START plan classifies a patient who has a radial pulse, respirations below 30/minute, and can follow simple commands as:

A. immediate.

B. delayed.

C. secondary.

D. minor.

© 2009 by Pearson Education, Inc. *First Responder*, Eighth Edition, Bergeron et al.

Determining Your Patient's Blood Pressure

APPENDIX

1

Reading Assignment: First Responder, 8th Edition, pages 569–575

NOTE: This material is optional in many Emergency Medical Responder courses. Your instructor will advise if the following will be included in your program.

KEY TERMS & DEFINITIONS

Define and explain the following terms from Appendix 1. Textbook page references are provided so that you can check your answers.

1. Describe the term **blood pressure** and explain its importance in patient assessment. (p. 569)

_____

_____

_____

_____

_____

_____

2. Explain the term **diastolic pressure**. (p. 569)

_____

_____

_____

_____

_____

3. Explain the term **systolic pressure**. (p. 569)

_____

_____

_____

© 2009 by Pearson Education, Inc. *First Responder*, Eighth Edition, Bergeron et al.

Appendix 1 Determining Your Patient's Blood Pressure **139**

_____

_____

4. Discuss the term **trending** as it relates to blood pressure and other vital signs. (p. 570)

_____

_____

_____

_____

EXERCISES

Complete the following exercises. Answers and/or textbook page references are provided at the back of the workbook. Before looking up your answers, think about your responses and discuss them with other students, Emergency Medical Responders, and emergency care providers.

INTRODUCTION

1. Explain why Emergency Medical Responders may take several blood pressure readings on any given patient. _____

_____

2. It is possible to estimate the systolic blood pressure of an adult male at rest. If the patient is 28 years old, his estimated systolic pressure would be _____.

3. A blood pressure reading above _____/_____ mmHg is considered high blood pressure.

MEASURING BLOOD PRESSURE

4. Describe how to place a blood pressure cuff on a patient's arm when taking a blood pressure reading.

_____

_____

_____

_____

5. Describe how to determine where to place the stethoscope on the patient's arm when taking a blood pressure reading

_____

_____

6. Explain the process of inflating the blood pressure cuff to the appropriate pressure. There are two methods.

   Method 1:

   _____

   _____

© 2009 by Pearson Education, Inc. *First Responder*, Eighth Edition, Bergeron et al.

Method 2:

_____

_____

7. Describe how to determine the systolic and diastolic pressures as you deflate the cuff.

_____

_____

_____

_____

_____

_____

8. Explain the steps of taking blood pressure by palpation.

_____

_____

_____

_____

_____

_____

_____

_____

9. List the reasons for taking blood pressure by palpation.

_____

_____

10. Give an example of how to record a blood pressure reading by palpation.

_____

PERSONAL DEVELOPMENT/APPLICATION

Mastering the skill of determining blood pressure takes a great deal of concentration and practice. Consider taking the following steps to improve this important skill:

- Take a blood pressure reading on THREE of your classmates using the auscultation method.
- Take a blood pressure reading on TWO of your classmates using the palpation method.
- If you have a blood pressure kit of your own, obtain readings of your family members or friends.
- Take one blood pressure every night of class and keep a log of the readings.

© 2009 by Pearson Education, Inc. *First Responder*, Eighth Edition, Bergeron et al.

APPENDIX 1 REVIEW

This self-test has been designed for you to take after you have completed the Reading Assignment, Key Terms & Definitions, and Exercises for Appendix 1. The answers and page references are given at the end of the workbook.

CIRCLE the letter of the correct answer to each question.

1. An adult may be in the later stages of shock if the systolic blood pressure is below:
   A. 90 mmHg.
   B. 100 mmHg.
   C. 110 mmHg.
   D. 120 mmHg.

2. A standard blood pressure cuff is typically used to obtain a blood pressure reading in the:
   A. carotid artery.
   B. brachial artery.
   C. ulnar vein.
   D. radial vein.

3. The blood pressure cuff must be inflated to a point that is _____ mmHg above the point where pulse sounds stop.
   A. 15
   B. 20
   C. 30
   D. 45

4. During the deflation of the cuff, the first "beating," or tapping, sounds heard indicate the _____ pressure.
   A. systolic
   B. pulse
   C. diastolic
   D. pulmonic

5. When the "beating," or tapping, sound fades and becomes dull or soft, this indicates the point of the _____ pressure.
   A. systolic
   B. pulse
   C. diastolic
   D. pulmonic

Breathing Aids and Oxygen Therapy

© 2009 by Pearson Education, Inc. *First Responder*, Eighth Edition, Bergeron et al.

Reading Assignment: First Responder, 8th Edition, pages 576–588

NOTE: This material is optional in many Emergency Medical Responder courses. Your instructor will advise you if the following will be covered in your course.

KEY TERMS & DEFINITIONS

Define and explain the following terms from Appendix 2. Textbook page references are provided so that you can check your answers.

1. What is a **bag-valve-mask (BVM) resuscitator** (also called a bag-valve-mask unit), and how is it used? (p. 586)

   _____

   _____

   _____

   _____

   _____

2. Explain the term **D cylinder.** (p. 578)

   _____

   _____

   _____

   _____

3. Define the term **flowmeter** and explain its purpose in oxygen delivery. (p. 581)

   _____

   _____

   _____

   _____

   _____

4. Compare and contrast the nasal cannula and the nonrebreather mask, stating the appropriate liter flow ranges for each. (pp. 581–583)

_____

_____

_____

_____

EXERCISES

Complete the following exercises. Answers and/or textbook page references are provided at the back of the workbook. Before looking up your answers, think about your responses and discuss them with other students, Emergency Medical Responders, and emergency care providers.

THE EMERGENCY MEDICAL RESPONDER'S ROLE

1. List FIVE responsibilities that come with the use of equipment in basic life support.

   A. _____

   B. _____

   C. _____

   D. _____

   E. _____

2. Explain why oxygen is considered a medication.

   _____

   _____

   _____

VENTILATION-ASSIST DEVICES

3. Name TWO devices that can be used to assist in the delivery of ventilations.

   A. _____

   B. _____

4. The bag-valve-mask resuscitator can deliver up to _____ % oxygen when attached to a supplemental oxygen supply.

5. Before using a bag-valve-mask resuscitator, should you insert an oropharyngeal airway? Explain your answer.

   _____

   _____

6. Describe the positioning of both hands when operating a bag-valve-mask unit by yourself.

_____

_____

_____

_____

_____

_____

7. For the adult patient who is not breathing, you should squeeze the bag once every
_____ seconds.

8. The greatest problem with the bag-valve-mask unit is a failure to form a proper
_____ between the mask and the patient's _____.

OXYGEN THERAPY

9. List at least FOUR advantages associated with the use of oxygen.

A. _____

B. _____

C. _____

D. _____

EQUIPMENT AND SUPPLIES FOR OXYGEN THERAPY

10. The oxygen in a full cylinder is kept at no less than _____ pounds per square
inch (PSI). It is brought to a safe working pressure by means of a _____
_____.

11. Oxygen is delivered in _____ per minute, which is regulated by a
_____.

12. Complete Table A2.1.

Table A2.1 Oxygen Delivery Devices

DEVICE	FLOW RATE	PERCENTAGE OF OXYGEN DELIVERED	SPECIAL USES
Nonrebreather Mask			
Nasal Cannula			

ADMINISTERING OXYGEN

13. List THREE devices, or adjuncts, that Emergency Medical Responders can use to deliver oxygen to a patient. (One of them may be considered an EMT-B level device.)

A. _____

B. _____

C. _____

14. Explain how the **demand valve** delivers oxygen.

_____

_____

_____

_____

15. List THREE standard features of a demand valve.

A. _____

B. _____

C. _____

PERSONAL DEVELOPMENT/APPLICATION

Administration of oxygen by Emergency Medical Responders may not be permitted in your system. Find out exactly what your local guidelines and medical direction procedures state regarding this skill. Also ask:

. . . your friends, family, and other laypersons about their perceptions about oxygen. How would they feel if it was necessary to wear a nonrebreather mask?

. . . if your workplace has oxygen on the premises and, if so, what type of cylinder is it? Where is it located? Become familiar with the system and assure that a system is in place to periodically check the tank.

APPENDIX 2 REVIEW

This self-test has been designed for you to take after you have completed the Reading Assignment, Key Terms & Definitions, and Exercises for Appendix 2. The answers and page references are given at the end of the workbook.

CIRCLE the letter of the correct answer to each question.

1. The bag-valve-mask resuscitator will deliver a maximum of _____ % of oxygen when attached to supplemental oxygen.
    A. 16
    B. 21
    C. 50
    D. 100

2. When ventilating the nonbreathing adult with a bag-valve-mask resuscitator, the bag should be squeezed once every _____ seconds.
    A. 2
    B. 5
    C. 10
    D. 15

3. The mask of a bag-valve-mask resuscitator should fit so that the:
    A. base is over the bridge of the nose and the apex is touching the chin.
    B. apex is over the bridge of the nose and the base rests between the lower lip and the projection of the chin.
    C. base is over the bridge of the nose and the apex rests between the lower lip and the projection of the chin.
    D. apex rests between the upper lip and the bridge of the nose and the base is over the projection of the chin.

4. More often than not, if the bag-valve-mask resuscitator will not deliver air to the patient's lungs, the problem is caused by:
    A. an improper seal between the patient's face and the mask.
    B. the bag is not being squeezed hard enough.
    C. the failure of a one-way valve.
    D. the patient is resisting or holding his breath.

5. When a pocket face mask is connected to an oxygen supply and is in place, air may be delivered to the patient by way of the oxygen supply and:
    A. mask ports.
    B. bag unit.
    C. bulb tube.
    D. the rescuer's breath.

Pharmacology

Reading Assignment: First Responder, 8th Edition, pages 589–599

NOTE: This material is optional in many Emergency Medical Responder courses. Your instructor will advise if this material will be included in your program, as well as which medications the Emergency Medical Responder is allowed to assist with based on your local protocols.

KEY TERMS & DEFINITIONS

Define and explain the following terms from Appendix 3. Textbook page references are provided so that you can check your answers.

1. Define the term **pharmacology**. (p. 589)

   _____

   _____

   _____

   _____

   _____

2. Define and give ONE example of each of the following terms. (p. 590)

   side effect

   _____

   _____

   _____

   _____

   _____

   indication

   _____

   _____

   _____

   _____

   _____

contraindication

_____

_____

_____

_____

_____

EXERCISES

Complete the following exercises. Answers and/or textbook page references are provided at the back of the workbook. Before looking up your answers, think about your responses and discuss them with other students, Emergency Medical Responders, and emergency care providers.

MEDICATIONS

1. Complete Table A3.1.

Table A3.1 Medications Carried on the Emergency Medical Responder Unit

NAME	INDICATION	IN YOUR OWN WORDS, HOW DOES IT WORK?
Activated Charcoal		
Oral Glucose		
Oxygen		

2. Match the following prescribed medications with their use.

_____ 1) Aerosol used to treat asthma	**A.**	Nitroglycerin
_____ 2) Dilates blood vessels	**B.**	Epinephrine auto-injectors
_____ 3) Used for allergic reactions	**C.**	Prescribed inhalers
_____ 4) Used for poisoning	**D.**	Oral glucose
_____ 5) Used for suspected low blood sugar	**E.**	Activated charcoal

3. Complete Table A3.2.

Table A3.2 Prescribed Medications

NAME	MEDICATION FORM	INDICATION	LIST TWO SIDE EFFECTS
Nitroglycerin			
Epinephrine Auto-Injectors			
Prescribed Inhalers			

4. List FIVE "rights" for giving any medication.

A. _____

B. _____

C. _____

D. _____

E. _____

5. List FIVE routes by which medication may be administered.

A. _____

B. _____

C. _____

D. _____

E. _____

6. Can Emergency Medical Responders give or assist with any medication without medical direction? Explain.

_____

_____

7. Discuss the term *transdermal* and list at least three common medications or types of medications that are administered in this manner.

_____

_____

_____

_____

PERSONAL DEVELOPMENT/APPLICATION

Using the information in Scans A3–1 through A3–5, create a set of "flash cards" out of 3 × 5 or 4 × 6 index cards. On one side, write the name of the medication; on the other side, list the indications, contraindications, side effects, and so on. Then, carry these cards with you wherever you go. You can quiz yourself or have others quiz you on a routine basis to learn the pharmacology of each medication.

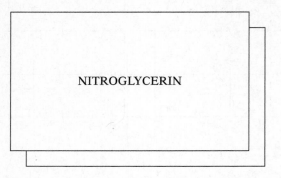

NITROGLYCERIN	

ACTION:	INDICATIONS:
FORM:	CONTRAINDICATIONS:
DOSAGE:	SIDE EFFECTS:
ADMINISTRATION:	

Next, think of scenarios in which the drugs discussed in Appendix 3 would be used. Discuss these situations with your fellow classmates.

APPENDIX 3 REVIEW

This self-test has been designed for you to take after you have completed the Reading Assignment, Key Terms & Definitions, and Exercises for Appendix 3. The answers and page references are given at the end of the workbook.

CIRCLE the letter of the correct answer to each question.

1. A responsive patient has ingested several bottles of pills along with vodka. Which of the following medications might be appropriate for this patient?
   A. syrup of ipecac
   B. nitroglycerin
   C. oral glucose
   D. activated charcoal

2. All of the following medications may be carried by Emergency Medical Responders EXCEPT:
   A. activated charcoal.
   B. oxygen.
   C. nitroglycerin.
   D. oral glucose.

3. Specific reasons or conditions for which a drug may be used are known as:
   A. actions.
   B. indications.
   C. contraindications.
   D. side effects.

4. Before assisting any patient with taking their own medication, an Emergency Medical Responder must:
   A. wait for ALS to arrive.
   B. locate the vial of life.
   C. ask the five "right" questions.
   D. have the patient sign a release.

5. When a drug is administered sublingually, this means it is:
   A. swallowed.
   B. placed under the tongue.
   C. injected into a muscle.
   D. inhaled, or breathed in.

Air Medical Operations

Reading Assignment: First Responder, 8th Edition, pages 600–604

NOTE: This material is optional in many Emergency Medical Responder courses. Your instructor will advise if this material will be included in your program.

KEY TERMS & DEFINITIONS

Define and explain the following terms from Appendix 4. Textbook page references are provided so that you can check your answers.

1. Define the term **scene call.** (p. 600)

   _____

   _____

   _____

   _____

2. Define the term **interfacility transport.** (p. 601)

   _____

   _____

   _____

   _____

3. List at least three common crew configurations for air medical transport. (p. 600)

   _____

   _____

   _____

EXERCISES

Complete the following exercises. Answers and/or textbook page references are provided at the back of the workbook. Before looking up your answers, think about your responses and discuss them with other students, Emergency Medical Responders, and emergency care providers.

1. Describe why a fixed wing (airplane) resource might be more appropriate than a rotor wing (helicopter) for an emergent transport.

    _____

    _____

    _____

2. Give an example of a situation where a rotor wing (helicopter) resource might be more appropriate than a fixed wing (airplane) for an emergent transport.

    _____

    _____

    _____

    _____

3. Provide THREE examples when a helicopter might be the most appropriate mode of transport.

    A. _____

    B. _____

    C. _____

4. Define the terms VFR and IFR and describe the differences between them.

    _____

    _____

    _____

5. List SEVEN characteristics of an appropriate helicopter landing zone:

    A. _____

    B. _____

    C. _____

    D. _____

    E. _____

    F. _____

    G. _____

PERSONAL DEVELOPMENT/APPLICATION

Many communities around the country are served by air medical resources. Some are privately owned and others are public entities. As a member of the EMS community you should be aware of these resources in your own community. Conduct some simple research into the availability of air medical resources in your area or an area close to you. Contact the service and obtain answers to the following questions:

1. How long has the program been in existence? _____

2. Is it private or public? _____

3. What type of aircraft do they fly—helicopters, airplanes, or both?

    _____

4. What type of crew configuration do they use?

    _____

5. Are they a VFR or IFR program? Both? _____

6. Do they respond to scene calls, interfacilities, or both?

    _____

Response to Terrorism and Weapons of Mass Destruction

Reading Assignment: First Responder, 8th Edition, pages 605–609

NOTE: This material is optional in many Emergency Medical Responder courses. Your instructor will advise if this material will be included in your program.

KEY TERMS & DEFINITIONS

Define and explain the following terms from Appendix 5. Textbook page references are provided so that you can check your answers.

1. Define the term **terrorism**. (p. 605)

   _____

   _____

   _____

   _____

2. List the two types of potential nuclear incidents. (p. 605)

   _____

   _____

   _____

   _____

3. List the three common categories of weapons of mass destruction. (pp. 605–608)

   _____

   _____

   _____

EXERCISES

Complete the following exercises. Answers and/or textbook page references are provided at the back of the workbook. Before looking up your answers, think about your responses and discuss them with other students, Emergency Medical Responders, and emergency care providers.

1. List the common signs and symptoms of exposure to each of the following agents:

    A. Nuclear/Radiological

    _____

    _____

    _____

    B. Biological

    _____

    _____

    _____

    C. Chemical

    _____

    _____

    _____

2. Describe the role of the Emergency Medical Responder who might be the first on the scene of a WMD incident. What signs might be present indicating such an event?

    _____

    _____

    _____

    _____

    _____

PERSONAL DEVELOPMENT/APPLICATION

Since the events of September 11, 2001, many communities and EMS systems have increased their preparedness for a WMD event. How has your EMS system or community increased its readiness for such an event? Have Emergency Medical Responders and other emergency personnel received specialized training or equipment? Contact your local EMS agency or someone involved in the local EMS system and ask these questions. Then bring their answers back to class with you and compare them with what others learned.

_____

_____

_____

_____

_____

© 2009 by Pearson Education, Inc. *First Responder*, Eighth Edition, Bergeron et al.

Swimming and Diving Incidents

Reading Assignment: First Responder, 8th Edition, pages 610–619

REMEMBER: Do only what you have been trained to do. Also, remember that mouth-to-mask techniques are not practical while the patient is in the water.

KEY TERMS & DEFINITIONS

Define and explain the following terms from Appendix 6. Textbook page references are provided so that you can check your answers.

1. Define the term **mammalian diving reflex** and explain how it may affect Emergency Medical Responder care. (p. 613)

    _____

    _____

    _____

    _____

    _____

    _____

2. Define the term **air embolism.** (p. 617)

    _____

    _____

    _____

    _____

3. Explain the concept of **decompression sickness,** or the "bends." (p. 617)

    _____

    _____

    _____

    _____

EXERCISES

Complete the following exercises. Answers and/or textbook page references are provided at the back of the workbook. Before looking up your answers, think about your responses and discuss them with other students, Emergency Medical Responders, and emergency care providers.

INCIDENTS INVOLVING THE WATER

1. List SIX problems an Emergency Medical Responder should look for when the patient is a victim of a water-related incident.

    A. _____

    B. _____

    C. _____

    D. _____

    E. _____

    F. _____

2. If the patient is responsive and close to the shore or poolside, hold out an object for him to grab and _____ him from the water. If he is too far away, _____ him an object that will _____. After this is done, you should try to find a way to _____ him from the water. Do NOT row or go into the water unless you are trained to do so.

CARE FOR THE PATIENT

3. In shallow-water incidents, always assume and provide care for _____.

4. In SEVEN steps, state what you should do to provide care for a responsive near-drowning victim who is out of the water when you arrive at the scene.

    A. _____

    B. _____

    C. _____

    D. _____

    E. _____

    F. _____

    G. _____

5. Can a cold-water drowning victim be resuscitated after being clinically dead for 20 minutes? _____ Explain.

    _____

    _____

6. You need to open the airway of an unresponsive near-drowning patient. What method should you use?

    _____

7. Is CPR thought to be effective if it is done while the patient is in the water? _____
   Explain.

   _____

   _____

DIVING INCIDENTS

8. List injuries to look for when assessing a victim of a diving-board incident.

   _____

   _____

   _____

9. If a scuba diver tries to hold his breath while under water, he runs a chance of developing a(n)
   _____ _____ in his blood.

10. List SEVEN signs of decompression sickness.

    A. _____

    B. _____

    C. _____

    D. _____

    E. _____

    F. _____

    G. _____

11. How should rescuers position a patient who may have decompression sickness? Why?

    _____

    _____

    _____

    _____

INCIDENTS INVOLVING ICE

12. List precautions to take and actions you should NOT do in an ice rescue situation.

    _____

    _____

    _____

    _____

    _____

13. You are at the scene of an ice incident and find EMS personnel involved in rescue and care. List SIX things you can do to help.

A. _____

B. _____

C. _____

D. _____

E. _____

F. _____

14. It is essential that the Emergency Medical Responder who is assisting with a water rescue always wear an appropriate _____.

PERSONAL DEVELOPMENT/APPLICATION

State some of the ways you as a member of the EMS system can improve your community's water safety record. How may you and your fellow Emergency Medical Responders use your "position" as members of the EMS system to influence the younger citizens where you live so that they will improve their own safety when near, on, or in the water?

_____

_____

_____

_____

_____

Are you prepared to handle water emergencies in your area? Explain how you or fellow Emergency Medical Responders can be trained to deal with this type of situation.

_____

_____

_____

_____

_____

_____

APPENDIX 6 REVIEW

This self-test has been designed for you to take after you have completed the Reading Assignment, Key Terms & Definitions, and Exercises for Appendix 6. The answers and page references are given at the end of the workbook.

CIRCLE the letter of the correct answer to each question.

1. An unresponsive patient is taken from the water. Your assessment shows that he is breathing and has a carotid pulse. You have to be on the alert for:

   A. shivering.
   B. rapid warming.
   C. mammalian diving reflex.
   D. hypothermia.

2. Which of the following represents the correct sequence of activities to be carried out by the Emergency Medical Responder attempting to rescue a responsive water incident victim?

   A. throw, tow, go
   B. pull, throw, tow
   C. throw, tow, row
   D. pull, throw, row

3. You wish to move a cold near-drowning patient to a warm place. The patient says that he can walk. You should:

   A. not allow him to walk.
   B. help him with a one-rescuer assist.
   C. encourage him to walk in order to help clear the lungs.
   D. suggest that he do some simple exercises before attempting to walk.

4. When providing mouth-to-mask resuscitation for an onshore, nonbreathing, near-drowning patient, you should:

   A. first pump the water from the lungs.
   B. use exactly the same techniques as you would for any nonbreathing patient.
   C. begin by forcing water from his stomach.
   D. expect more resistance to your efforts to ventilate.

5. You should open the airway of an unwitnessed, unresponsive near-drowning patient by using the _____ maneuver.

   A. head-tilt, chin-lift
   B. head-tilt, neck-lift
   C. jaw-thrust
   D. slight head-tilt

Posttest

This is a posttest. It has been designed for you to take after you have completed the last unit in your Emergency Medical Responder course. This test is provided for self-evaluation so that you can see your weaknesses before taking a final exam. Text page references are provided so that you can go back and restudy problem areas before final testing.

Because this is a posttest, take as much time as needed to complete it. Your best approach would be to set aside one solid hour for the test. Answers are provided so you can check your test and note the pages you need to reread and study.

CIRCLE the letter of the correct answer to each question.

1. An injured adult patient wants you to help him. He starts calling you "doctor." You should tell him you are an Emergency Medical Responder trained in emergency care so that his consent is:
   A. implied.
   B actual.
   C. informed.
   D. limited.

2. A penetrating wound to the upper-right quadrant of the abdomen will likely cause injury to the:
   A. spleen.
   B. liver.
   C. urinary bladder.
   D. appendix.

3. You arrive at the scene where a young man fell from the roof of a house. You find him to be unresponsive. You should first:
   A. ensure an open airway.
   B. begin mouth-to-mask resuscitation.
   C. take a carotid pulse.
   D. perform a complete patient assessment.

4. During the patient assessment, checking for abdominal tenderness is done after assessing the:
   A. back.
   B. abdomen.
   C. pelvis.
   D. the chest.

5. For the adult patient, the rate of ventilations during mouth-to-mask resuscitation is:
   A. one every 5–6 seconds.
   B. one every 15 seconds.
   C. two every 5–6 seconds.
   D. two every 15 seconds.

© 2009 by Pearson Education, Inc. *First Responder*, Eighth Edition, Bergeron et al.

6. During single-rescuer CPR for the adult patient, compressions and ventilations are provided at a ratio of _____ breath(s) every _____ compressions at a rate of _____ compressions per minute.

   A. 1, 30, 50
   B. 1, 5, 80
   C. 2, 30, 100
   D. 2, 15, 100

7. The order of care when trying to control severe bleeding is:

   A. elevation, direct pressure, pressure points.
   B. pressure points, direct pressure, elevation.
   C. direct pressure, elevation, pressure points.
   D. pressure points, direct pressure, elevation.

8. When caring for a patient without a head or spinal injury who is developing shock, you should:

   A. elevate the head.
   B. elevate the feet.
   C. elevate the upper body.
   D. leave in a flat position.

9. If you provide emergency care in good faith, to the best of your ability, you are protected in most states by _____ laws.

   A. actual consent
   B. Good Samaritan
   C. implied consent
   D. applied consent

10. In two-rescuer CPR for the adult patient, ventilations and compressions are delivered at a ratio and rate of:

    A. one breath every 5 compressions and 60 to 80 compressions per minute.
    B. one breath every 5 compressions and 100 compressions per minute.
    C. two breaths every 30 compressions and 100 compressions per minute.
    D two breaths every 15 compressions and 80 compressions per minute.

11. A patient has an object impaled in the eye. You should:

    A. remove the object and apply direct pressure with a gauze pad.
    B. remove the object and apply a loose dressing.
    C. leave the object in place, pad around the eye, and place a cup or cone over the object.
    D. leave the object in place, apply a pressure dressing around the object, and place a cup or cone over the object.

12. An unresponsive person is found in a field. He has periods of responsiveness, but he remains unresponsive to verbal stimuli during these intervals. His face is swollen and blotchy; respirations are labored and wheezing. His pulse is very weak. Your care should focus on the possibility of:

    A. abdominal injury.
    B. heat emergency.
    C. diabetic emergency.
    D. anaphylactic shock.

13. In the adult patient, the CPR compression site is:

    A. directly below the nipples.
    B. two finger-widths below the collarbones, along the midline of the body.
    C. over the lower half of the sternum.
    D. three finger-widths to the right of the left nipple.

14. When providing single-rescuer CPR for a child, breaths and compressions are provided at a ratio and rate of:

   A. one breath every 5 compressions at a rate of 60 compressions per minute.
   B. one breath every 5 compressions at a rate of 100 compressions per minute.
   C. two breaths every 30 compressions at a rate of 100 compressions per minute.
   D. two breaths every 30 compressions at a rate of 80 compressions per minute.

15. When providing emergency care that does not require ventilating the patient, your best defense against most infectious diseases is to:

   A. wear a gauze mask.
   B. use occlusive dressings.
   C. wear latex or vinyl gloves.
   D. wash your hands with bleach after touching blood or body fluids.

16. The term "body substance isolation" may best be defined as:

   A. taking precautions around a patient who is bleeding.
   B. warning other rescuers when a patient has a disease.
   C. protecting yourself from all body fluids.
   D. isolating any patient who may have an infectious disease.

17. A patient has an open wound of the abdomen and his intestines have been exposed. You should:

   A. apply a moist sterile dressing over the exposed organs.
   B. push the intestine back into the abdominal cavity.
   C. apply direct pressure.
   D. place a dry sterile dressing over the exposed organs.

18. A patient has clear fluids draining from his ear. You should:

   A. pack the ear canal.
   B. apply a pressure dressing.
   C. do nothing.
   D. cover the ear with a loose dressing.

19. It is recommended that all Emergency Medical Responders receive a vaccination for:

   A. HIV.
   B. meningitis.
   C. tuberculosis.
   D. hepatitis B.

20. When providing mouth-to-mask ventilations for a patient with a suspected spinal injury, you should use the _____ maneuver to open the airway.

   A. jaw-thrust
   B. head-tilt, neck-lift
   C. head-tilt, chin-lift
   D. neutral neck position

21. You find dark, red blood flowing from a neck wound. As soon as practical after applying direct pressure, you should:

   A. apply a tourniquet.
   B. use the carotid artery pressure point.
   C. apply an occlusive dressing.
   D. apply a bulky dressing.

22. As you approach the victim of a fall, you note that he is not responsive. The patient is lying face up with both arms pulled tight against his chest. You should suspect possible:

   A. severe internal bleeding.
   B. spinal injury.
   C. pelvic fractures.
   D. hip dislocation.

23. When caring for an open wound, your first step is to:
   A. cover the wound.
   B. clean the site.
   C. control bleeding.
   D. prevent contamination.

24. When caring for an injured eye, you should:
   A. apply direct pressure.
   B. apply a pressure dressing.
   C. cover both eyes.
   D. leave both eyes open.

25. An object is loosely impaled in the cheek. Its point has broken through the cheek wall into the mouth. You should:
   A. remove the object and carefully place packs between teeth and cheek wall.
   B. not remove the object but place packs between the teeth and cheek wall.
   C. simply remove the object.
   D. leave the object in place.

26. Geriatric patients are often less able to defend against illness and may take much longer to recover when they do become ill. This often results in:
   A. multiple simultaneous illnesses.
   B. forgetting doctor appointments.
   C. taking the wrong medications.
   D. hearing loss.

27. When breathing and circulation stop, irreversible damage in the patient's brain is likely to begin within:
   A. 30 seconds.
   B. 1 to 3 minutes.
   C. 4 to 6 minutes.
   D. 10 to 15 minutes.

28. A patient has an object impaled in the chest. You should:
   A. do nothing to the site.
   B. stabilize the object with pads of dressing.
   C. remove the object and apply an occlusive dressing.
   D. remove the object and apply a trauma dressing.

29. A patient has an obvious sucking chest wound. You should:
   A. apply an occlusive dressing.
   B. apply a cravat.
   C. apply a trauma dressing.
   D. wait for the next level of care.

30. At the scene of a hazardous materials incident, the safe zone should be established:
   A. downhill and upwind.
   B. uphill and upwind.
   C. uphill and downwind.
   D. downhill and downwind.

31. The loss of mobility is a common complaint among the elderly and can lead to other problems such as:
   A. better nutrition.
   B. independence.
   C. depression.
   D. nearsightedness.

32. A responsive patient has a minor closed-head injury, with no indications of spinal injury. This patient should be positioned:
   A. as found.
   B. with legs elevated.
   C. face down.
   D. with upper body elevated.

33. When assessing a geriatric patient who has an altered mental status, you must:
    A. do your best to keep him awake and alert.
    B. determine if his mental state is normal.
    C. determine if he has had any recent surgeries.
    D. find out from family if he can walk or not.

34. A patient is very restless and complains of pain in his chest. His breathing is very labored. You should care for this patient as though he may be experiencing:
    A. a stroke (CVA).
    B. congestive heart failure.
    C. a heart attack.
    D. an epileptic seizure.

35. A patient is having difficulty breathing. He must be moved quickly from the second floor of his house to a waiting ambulance. Which device would work best for this move?
    A. scoop stretcher
    B. stair chair
    C. short spine board
    D. basket stretcher

36. A patient has labored, rapid breathing. His ankles are swollen. You note a blue discoloration to his lips. The patient insists upon sitting up and supporting his upper body weight on his elbows. You should suspect:
    A. congestive heart failure.
    B. mild epilepsy.
    C. insulin shock.
    D. stroke (CVA).

37. A patient with an altered mental status shows signs and symptoms of possible stroke. He should be positioned:
    A. face down.
    B. as found.
    C. with legs elevated.
    D. in the recovery position.

38. The aging process can cause a degeneration of the heart's electrical system, which can lead to:
    a. hearing loss.
    b. vision loss.
    c. dysrhythmias.
    d. stroke (brain attack).

39. At the scene of a collapsed building, a rescuer crawls into the wreckage and finds two victims. The first patient is responsive and doing okay. The second patient appears to have stopped breathing. In order to get to the second patient, the rescuer may have to perform a(n):
    A. emergency move.
    B. direct-ground lift.
    C. nonemergency move.
    D. extremity lift.

40. When performing rescue breathing for an infant, breaths are delivered at the rate of:
    A. one every second.
    B. one every 3–5 seconds.
    C. one every 9 seconds.
    D. two every 5–6 seconds.

41. A woman's first labor normally lasts at least _____ hour(s).
    A. 1   B. 4   C. 8   D. 16

42. During a breech birth, the baby's head must deliver within 3 minutes of its buttocks and trunk. If delivery of the head does not occur in this time period, you should:
    A. transport immediately.
    B. wait 5 minutes as you massage the mother's abdomen.
    C. insert your fingers into the mother's vagina and create an airway for the baby.
    D. wait for the next level of care to arrive.

© 2009 by Pearson Education, Inc. *First Responder*, Eighth Edition, Bergeron et al.

43. To control normal postdelivery vaginal bleeding, you should place a sanitary pad over the mother's vaginal opening, place her legs together, elevate her legs, and:

A. massage her abdomen over the site of the uterus (womb).
B. apply direct pressure over the pad.
C. have her use her thighs to tighten and release pressure on the napkin.
D. have her apply direct pressure over the pad.

44. If a newborn does not start breathing on his own within 30 seconds, you should:

A. massage the mother's abdomen.
B. tap your fingers on the soles of the baby's feet or vigorously rub his back.
C. hold the baby up by his ankles and slap the buttocks.
D. tie off the umbilical cord.

45. When caring for a patient who has been exposed to a dry powder chemical, you should:

A. soak the site in cold water for 5 minutes.
B. wash the site in warm water for 15 minutes.
C. wash the site and apply a burn ointment.
D. brush away the powder before washing the site.

46. A suspected overdose patient is very sleepy. His pulse and breathing rates are dangerously low. You note that his pupils are constricted and he is sweating heavily. The patient has probably overdosed on:

A. uppers.
B. downers.
C. narcotics.
D. volatile chemicals.

47. You are caring for a responsive 2-year-old patient who has ingested an unknown amount of cough syrup. You have called for medical direction, which is likely to advise which of the following emergency care procedures?

A. Induce vomiting with syrup of ipecac.
B. Give the patient mineral oil to drink.
C. Induce vomiting with activated charcoal and water.
D. Dilute the poison by having the patient drink water or milk.

48. Age-related changes in the musculoskeletal system can lead to changes in posture, range of motion, and:

A. awareness.
B. medication usage.
C. mental status.
D. balance.

49. For patients having behavioral emergencies, you should:

A. tell them that everything is fine and not to worry.
B. tell them they are to listen to you and do what you say because you are there to help.
C. tell them that you are trained to care for people having behavioral emergencies.
D. talk to these patients and let them know that you are listening to what they tell you.

50. In the START triage system, which of the following patients would be considered in the "Immediate" (Priority 1) category?

A. A responsive burn victim.
B. An unresponsive female with moderate bleeding.
C. A responsive child with extremity injuries.
D. An adult male in cardiac arrest.

Reference Section

The following pages contain the flow-of-care diagrams that are also found in the student text. They are placed here for your further reference. The contents below will help you locate individual diagrams.

Remember: Flow Diagrams are learning tools. They are not complete protocols or lists of every step in assessment and care for every situation seen in First Responder-level emergency care.

FLOW-OF-CARE DIAGRAMS

© 2009 by Pearson Education, Inc. *First Responder*, Eighth Edition, Bergeron et al.

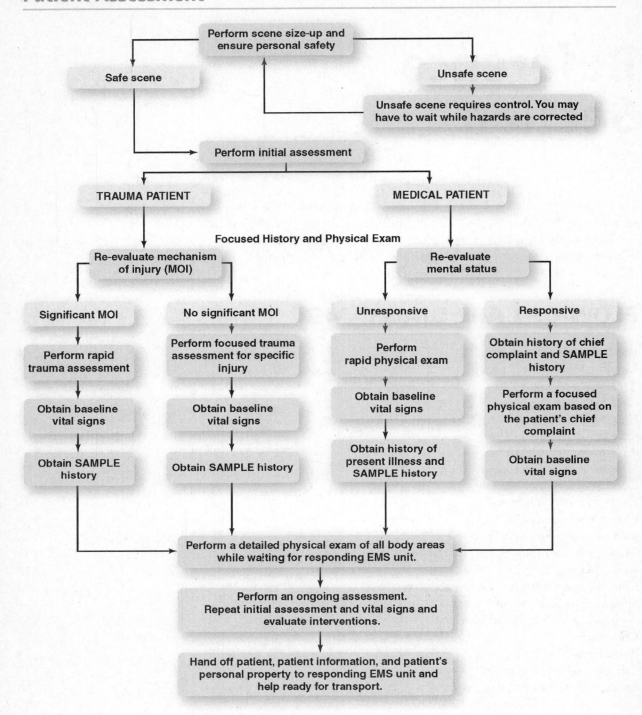

Perform scene size-up and ensure personal safety

Safe scene

Unsafe scene

Unsafe scene requires control. You may have to wait while hazards are corrected

Perform initial assessment

TRAUMA PATIENT

MEDICAL PATIENT

Focused History and Physical Exam

Re-evaluate mechanism of injury (MOI)

Re-evaluate mental status

Significant MOI

No significant MOI

Unresponsive

Responsive

Perform rapid trauma assessment

Perform focused trauma assessment for specific injury

Perform rapid physical exam

Obtain history of chief complaint and SAMPLE history

Obtain baseline vital signs

Obtain baseline vital signs

Obtain baseline vital signs

Perform a focused physical exam based on the patient's chief complaint

Obtain SAMPLE history

Obtain SAMPLE history

Obtain history of present illness and SAMPLE history

Obtain baseline vital signs

Perform a detailed physical exam of all body areas while waiting for responding EMS unit.

Perform an ongoing assessment. Repeat initial assessment and vital signs and evaluate interventions.

Hand off patient, patient information, and patient's personal property to responding EMS unit and help ready for transport.

Care for Medical Emergencies

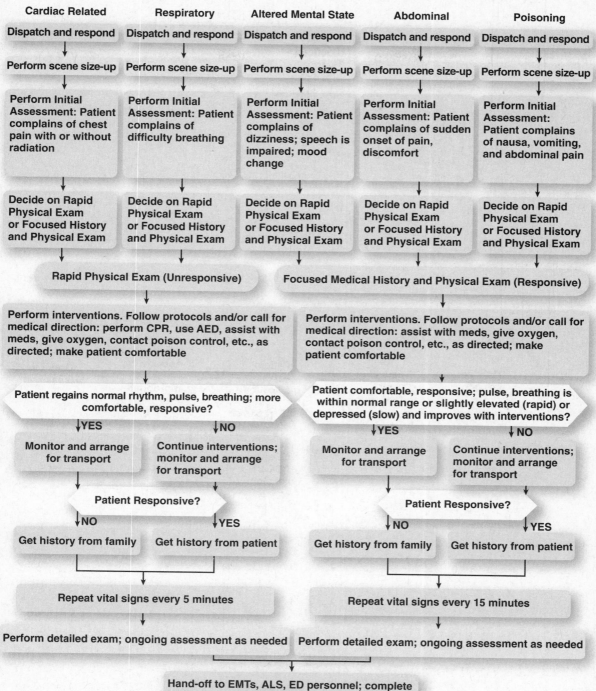

Cardiac Related

Dispatch and respond

Perform scene size-up

Perform Initial Assessment: Patient complains of chest pain with or without radiation

Decide on Rapid Physical Exam or Focused History and Physical Exam

Respiratory

Dispatch and respond

Perform scene size-up

Perform Initial Assessment: Patient complains of difficulty breathing

Decide on Rapid Physical Exam or Focused History and Physical Exam

Altered Mental State

Dispatch and respond

Perform scene size-up

Perform Initial Assessment: Patient complains of dizziness; speech is impaired; mood change

Decide on Rapid Physical Exam or Focused History and Physical Exam

Abdominal

Dispatch and respond

Perform scene size-up

Perform Initial Assessment: Patient complains of sudden onset of pain, discomfort

Decide on Rapid Physical Exam or Focused History and Physical Exam

Poisoning

Dispatch and respond

Perform scene size-up

Perform Initial Assessment: Patient complains of nausa, vomiting, and abdominal pain

Decide on Rapid Physical Exam or Focused History and Physical Exam

Rapid Physical Exam (Unresponsive)

Focused Medical History and Physical Exam (Responsive)

Perform interventions. Follow protocols and/or call for medical direction: perform CPR, use AED, assist with meds, give oxygen, contact poison control, etc., as directed; make patient comfortable

Perform interventions. Follow protocols and/or call for medical direction: assist with meds, give oxygen, contact poison control, etc., as directed; make patient comfortable

Patient regains normal rhythm, pulse, breathing; more comfortable, responsive?

↓YES — Monitor and arrange for transport
↓NO — Continue interventions; monitor and arrange for transport

Patient comfortable, responsive; pulse, breathing is within normal range or slightly elevated (rapid) or depressed (slow) and improves with interventions?

↓YES — Monitor and arrange for transport
↓NO — Continue interventions; monitor and arrange for transport

Patient Responsive?

↓NO — Get history from family
↓YES — Get history from patient

Patient Responsive?

↓NO — Get history from family
↓YES — Get history from patient

Repeat vital signs every 5 minutes

Repeat vital signs every 15 minutes

Perform detailed exam; ongoing assessment as needed

Perform detailed exam; ongoing assessment as needed

Hand-off to EMTs, ALS, ED personnel; complete reports; prepare for next response

Assessment of Chest Pain

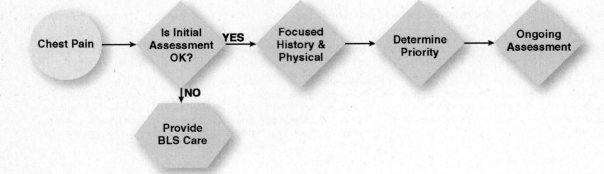

Care for Chest Pain

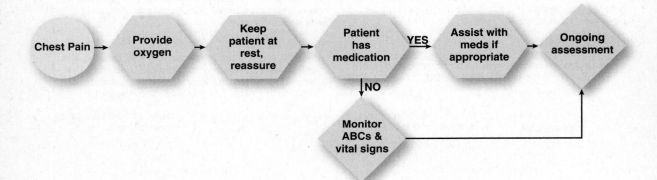

Care for Respiratory Distress

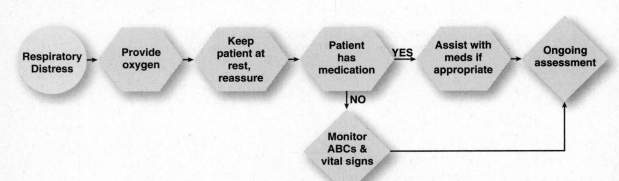

Care for Abdominal Pain

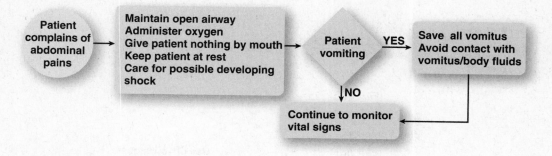

Patient complains of abdominal pains → Maintain open airway / Administer oxygen / Give patient nothing by mouth / Keep patient at rest / Care for possible developing shock → Patient vomiting — YES → Save all vomitus / Avoid contact with vomitus/body fluids

Patient vomiting — NO → Continue to monitor vital signs

Assessment of a Heat Emergency

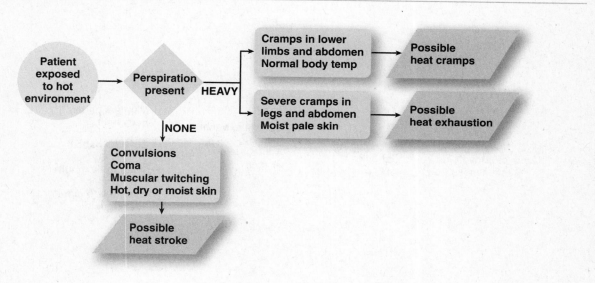

Patient exposed to hot environment → Perspiration present — HEAVY → Cramps in lower limbs and abdomen / Normal body temp → Possible heat cramps

Severe cramps in legs and abdomen / Moist pale skin → Possible heat exhaustion

Perspiration present — NONE → Convulsions / Coma / Muscular twitching / Hot, dry or moist skin → Possible heat stroke

Care for a Heat Emergency

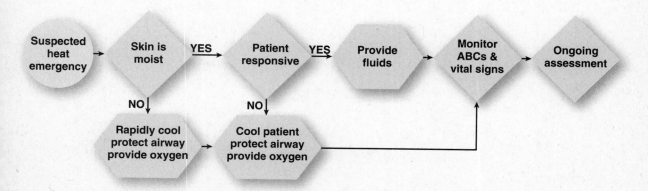

Suspected heat emergency → Skin is moist — YES → Patient responsive — YES → Provide fluids → Monitor ABCs & vital signs → Ongoing assessment

Skin is moist — NO → Rapidly cool / protect airway / provide oxygen

Patient responsive — NO → Cool patient / protect airway / provide oxygen

© 2009 by Pearson Education, Inc. *First Responder*, Eighth Edition, Bergeron et al.

Control of External Bleeding

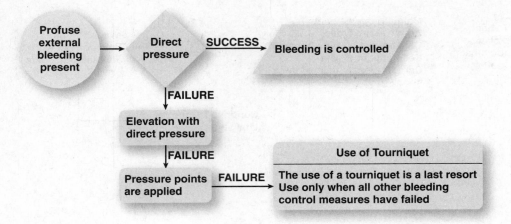

Profuse external bleeding present → **Direct pressure** — SUCCESS → **Bleeding is controlled**

Direct pressure ↓ FAILURE → **Elevation with direct pressure** ↓ FAILURE → **Pressure points are applied** — FAILURE →

Use of Tourniquet
The use of a tourniquet is a last resort
Use only when all other bleeding control measures have failed

Care of Developing Shock

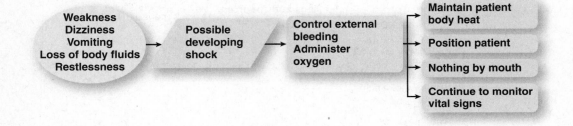

**Weakness
Dizziness
Vomiting
Loss of body fluids
Restlessness** → **Possible developing shock** → **Control external bleeding
Administer oxygen** →

- **Maintain patient body heat**
- **Position patient**
- **Nothing by mouth**
- **Continue to monitor vital signs**

Care for Soft-Tissue Injuries

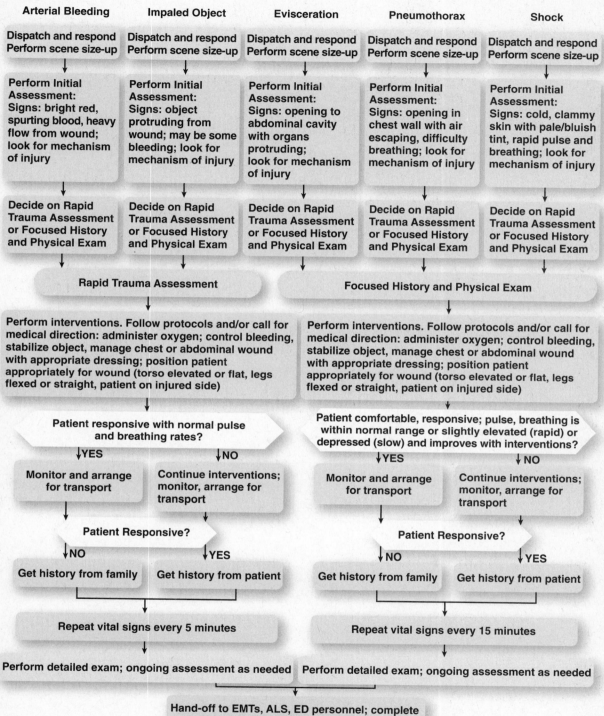

Arterial Bleeding	Impaled Object	Evisceration	Pneumothorax	Shock
Dispatch and respond Perform scene size-up	Dispatch and respond Perform scene size-up	Dispatch and respond Perform scene size-up	Dispatch and respond Perform scene size-up	Dispatch and respond Perform scene size-up
Perform Initial Assessment: Signs: bright red, spurting blood, heavy flow from wound; look for mechanism of injury	Perform Initial Assessment: Signs: object protruding from wound; may be some bleeding; look for mechanism of injury	Perform Initial Assessment: Signs: opening to abdominal cavity with organs protruding; look for mechanism of injury	Perform Initial Assessment: Signs: opening in chest wall with air escaping, difficulty breathing; look for mechanism of injury	Perform Initial Assessment: Signs: cold, clammy skin with pale/bluish tint, rapid pulse and breathing; look for mechanism of injury
Decide on Rapid Trauma Assessment or Focused History and Physical Exam	Decide on Rapid Trauma Assessment or Focused History and Physical Exam	Decide on Rapid Trauma Assessment or Focused History and Physical Exam	Decide on Rapid Trauma Assessment or Focused History and Physical Exam	Decide on Rapid Trauma Assessment or Focused History and Physical Exam

Rapid Trauma Assessment

Focused History and Physical Exam

Perform interventions. Follow protocols and/or call for medical direction: administer oxygen; control bleeding, stabilize object, manage chest or abdominal wound with appropriate dressing; position patient appropriately for wound (torso elevated or flat, legs flexed or straight, patient on injured side)

Perform interventions. Follow protocols and/or call for medical direction: administer oxygen; control bleeding, stabilize object, manage chest or abdominal wound with appropriate dressing; position patient appropriately for wound (torso elevated or flat, legs flexed or straight, patient on injured side)

Patient responsive with normal pulse and breathing rates?

↓YES → Monitor and arrange for transport

↓NO → Continue interventions; monitor, arrange for transport

Patient comfortable, responsive; pulse, breathing is within normal range or slightly elevated (rapid) or depressed (slow) and improves with interventions?

↓YES → Monitor and arrange for transport

↓NO → Continue interventions; monitor, arrange for transport

Patient Responsive?

↓NO → Get history from family

↓YES → Get history from patient

Patient Responsive?

↓NO → Get history from family

↓YES → Get history from patient

Repeat vital signs every 5 minutes

Repeat vital signs every 15 minutes

Perform detailed exam; ongoing assessment as needed

Perform detailed exam; ongoing assessment as needed

Hand-off to EMTs, ALS, ED personnel; complete reports; prepare for next response

© 2009 by Pearson Education, Inc. *First Responder*, Eighth Edition, Bergeron et al.

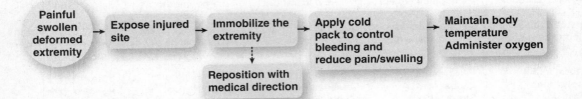

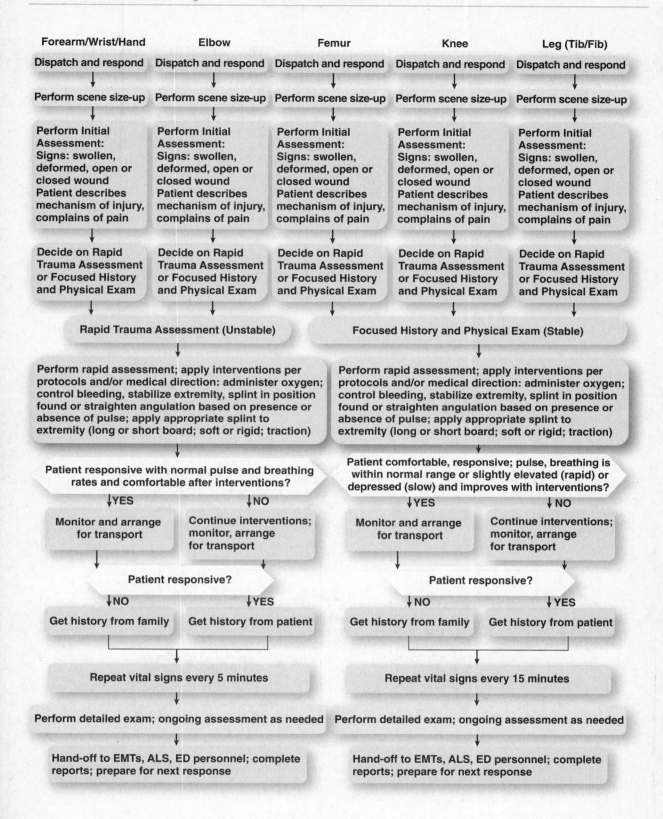

Forearm/Wrist/Hand	Elbow	Femur	Knee	Leg (Tib/Fib)
Dispatch and respond	Dispatch and respond	Dispatch and respond	Dispatch and respond	Dispatch and respond
Perform scene size-up	Perform scene size-up	Perform scene size-up	Perform scene size-up	Perform scene size-up

Perform Initial Assessment: Signs: swollen, deformed, open or closed wound. Patient describes mechanism of injury, complains of pain

Decide on Rapid Trauma Assessment or Focused History and Physical Exam

Rapid Trauma Assessment (Unstable)

Focused History and Physical Exam (Stable)

Perform rapid assessment; apply interventions per protocols and/or medical direction: administer oxygen; control bleeding, stabilize extremity, splint in position found or straighten angulation based on presence or absence of pulse; apply appropriate splint to extremity (long or short board; soft or rigid; traction)

Patient responsive with normal pulse and breathing rates and comfortable after interventions?

YES → Monitor and arrange for transport

NO → Continue interventions; monitor, arrange for transport

Patient responsive?

NO → Get history from family

YES → Get history from patient

Repeat vital signs every 5 minutes

Patient comfortable, responsive; pulse, breathing is within normal range or slightly elevated (rapid) or depressed (slow) and improves with interventions?

YES → Monitor and arrange for transport

NO → Continue interventions; monitor, arrange for transport

Patient responsive?

NO → Get history from family

YES → Get history from patient

Repeat vital signs every 15 minutes

Perform detailed exam; ongoing assessment as needed

Hand-off to EMTs, ALS, ED personnel; complete reports; prepare for next response

Care of Upper Extremity Injuries

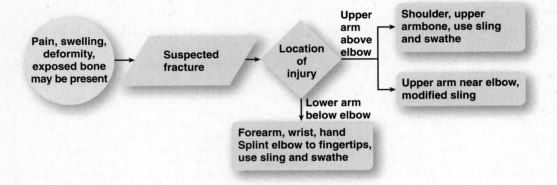

Pain, swelling, deformity, exposed bone may be present → **Suspected fracture** → **Location of injury**

- Upper arm above elbow → **Shoulder, upper armbone, use sling and swathe**
- → **Upper arm near elbow, modified sling**
- Lower arm below elbow → **Forearm, wrist, hand Splint elbow to fingertips, use sling and swathe**

Care of Lower Extremity Injuries

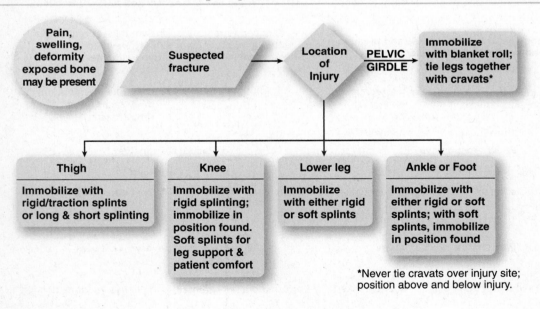

Pain, swelling, deformity exposed bone may be present → **Suspected fracture** → **Location of Injury**

PELVIC GIRDLE → **Immobilize with blanket roll; tie legs together with cravats***

Thigh	Knee	Lower leg	Ankle or Foot
Immobilize with rigid/traction splints or long & short splinting	Immobilize with rigid splinting; immobilize in position found. Soft splints for leg support & patient comfort	Immobilize with either rigid or soft splints	Immobilize with either rigid or soft splints; with soft splints, immobilize in position found

*Never tie cravats over injury site; position above and below injury.

Spinal Injury Assessment

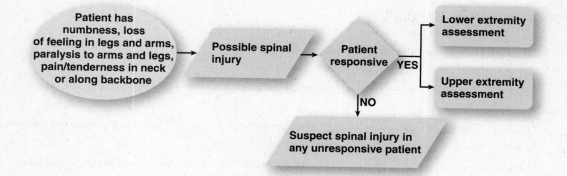

- Patient has numbness, loss of feeling in legs and arms, paralysis to arms and legs, pain/tenderness in neck or along backbone → Possible spinal injury → Patient responsive
  - YES → Lower extremity assessment / Upper extremity assessment
  - NO → Suspect spinal injury in any unresponsive patient

Assisting in a Normal Delivery

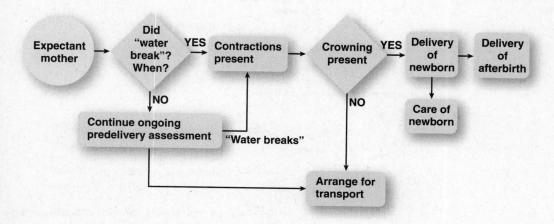

- Expectant mother → Did "water break"? When?
  - YES → Contractions present → Crowning present
    - YES → Delivery of newborn → Delivery of afterbirth; Care of newborn
    - NO → Arrange for transport
  - NO → Continue ongoing predelivery assessment → "Water breaks" → Contractions present; Arrange for transport

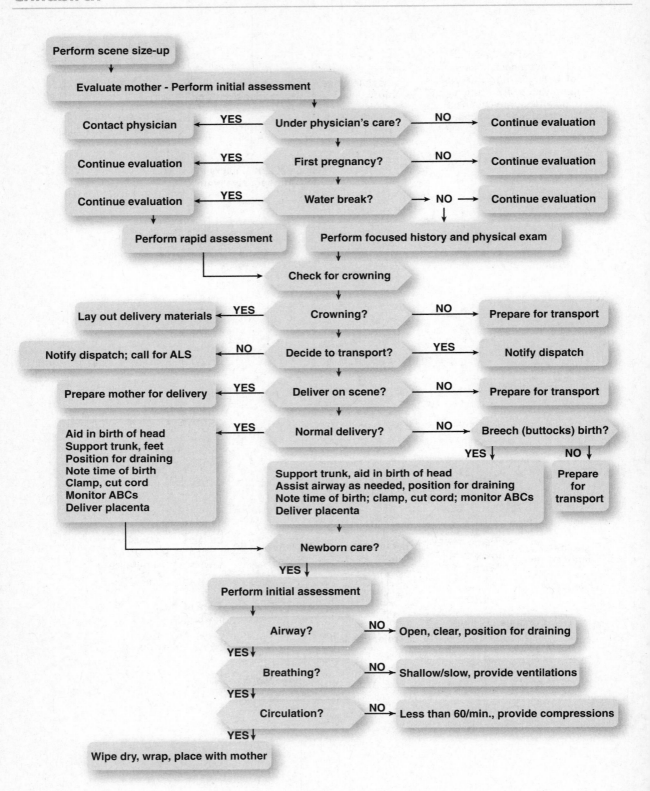

Assessment of the Newborn

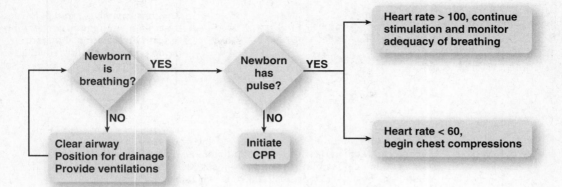

Complications of Childbirth

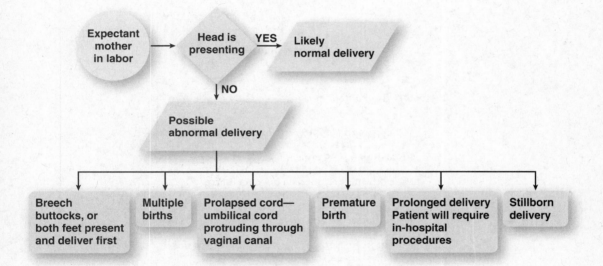

© 2009 by Pearson Education, Inc. *First Responder*, Eighth Edition, Bergeron et al.

Respond to an 11 year-old-boy who is in the school nurse's office with trouble breathing → Scene size-up; Initial assessment → Signs: responsive, rapid pulse and breathing, sitting up-right, leaning forward on his arms, agitated; blood pressure slightly elevated

Focused physical exam (responsive)

Perform interventions. Follow protocols and/or call for medical direction: provide oxygen (humidified, if possible or as soon as possible) via bag-valve-mask; keep patient as calm as possible; call dispatch for ALS assistance and rapid transport. Assist with medication if trained and protocols allow.

Pulse and breathing stabilize (within normal range) Emotional state improves

NO↓   ↓YES

Continue interventions

Is child able to give history

NO↓   ↓YES

Get history from nurse/family   Get history from patient

S - signs and symptoms (How long has child been wheezing?)
A - allergies (Any known allergies to drugs, food, pollens, inhalants, pet dander?)
M - medications (Does he have an inhaler for asthma attacks, has he used it, how frequently?)
P - pertinent past history (Has he had a recent cold or respiratory infection?)
L - last meal/food eaten (Has he had any fluids since this attack started?)
E - events leading to calling 911 (What was he doing or exposed to that may have caused the attack?)

Repeat vital signs every 5 minutes

Perform detailed exam (toe-to-head, if necessary) and ongoing assessment while waiting for transport personnel.

Hand off to EMTs, ALS; complete reports; prepare for next response

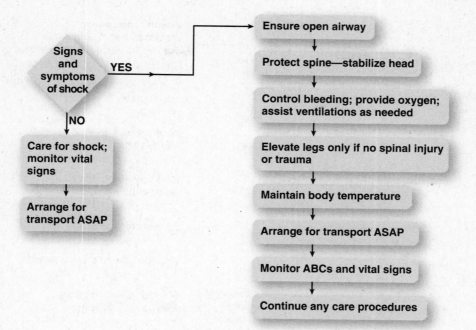

Signs and symptoms of shock

YES → Ensure open airway ↓ Protect spine—stabilize head ↓ Control bleeding; provide oxygen; assist ventilations as needed ↓ Elevate legs only if no spinal injury or trauma ↓ Maintain body temperature ↓ Arrange for transport ASAP ↓ Monitor ABCs and vital signs ↓ Continue any care procedures

NO ↓ Care for shock; monitor vital signs ↓ Arrange for transport ASAP

© 2009 by Pearson Education, Inc. *First Responder*, Eighth Edition, Bergeron et al.

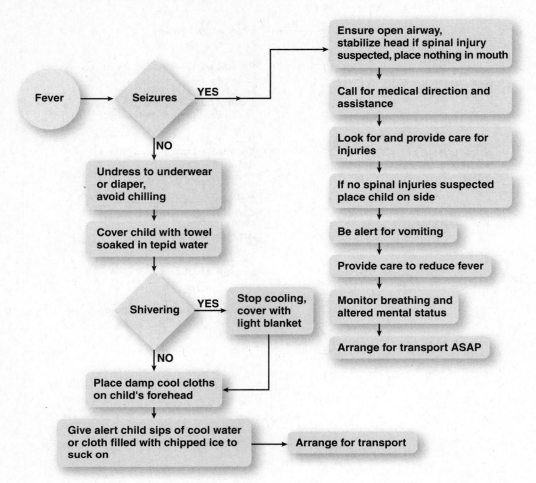

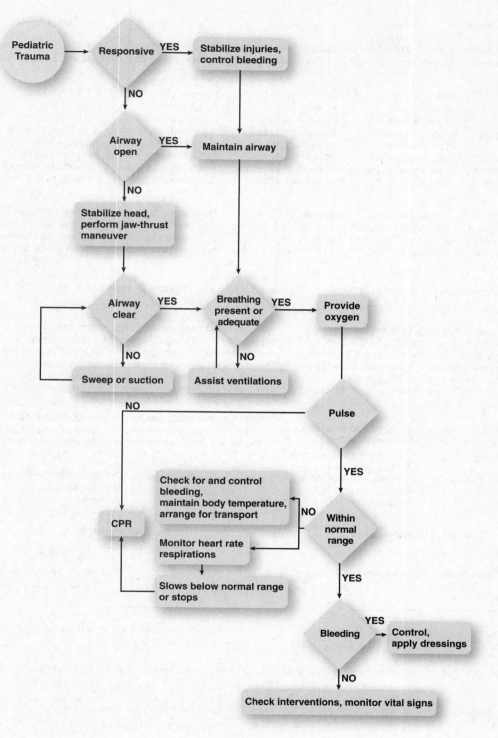

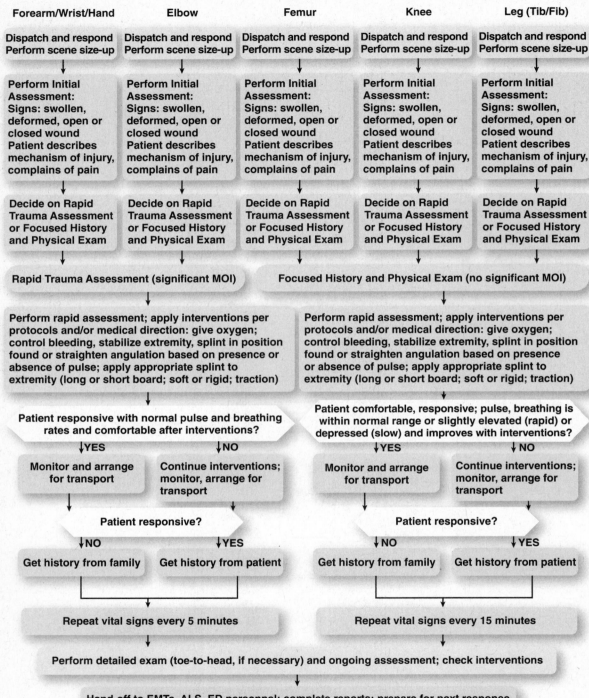

Forearm/Wrist/Hand	Elbow	Femur	Knee	Leg (Tib/Fib)
Dispatch and respond Perform scene size-up	Dispatch and respond Perform scene size-up	Dispatch and respond Perform scene size-up	Dispatch and respond Perform scene size-up	Dispatch and respond Perform scene size-up

Perform Initial Assessment: Signs: swollen, deformed, open or closed wound Patient describes mechanism of injury, complains of pain

Decide on Rapid Trauma Assessment or Focused History and Physical Exam

Rapid Trauma Assessment (significant MOI) — **Focused History and Physical Exam (no significant MOI)**

Perform rapid assessment; apply interventions per protocols and/or medical direction: give oxygen; control bleeding, stabilize extremity, splint in position found or straighten angulation based on presence or absence of pulse; apply appropriate splint to extremity (long or short board; soft or rigid; traction)

Patient responsive with normal pulse and breathing rates and comfortable after interventions?

↓YES → Monitor and arrange for transport

↓NO → Continue interventions; monitor, arrange for transport

Patient comfortable, responsive; pulse, breathing is within normal range or slightly elevated (rapid) or depressed (slow) and improves with interventions?

↓YES → Monitor and arrange for transport

↓NO → Continue interventions; monitor, arrange for transport

Patient responsive?

↓NO → Get history from family

↓YES → Get history from patient

Repeat vital signs every 5 minutes

Repeat vital signs every 15 minutes

Perform detailed exam (toe-to-head, if necessary) and ongoing assessment; check interventions

Hand-off to EMTs, ALS, ED personnel; complete reports; prepare for next response

Pediatric Bleeding, Shock, and Soft-Tissue Injuries

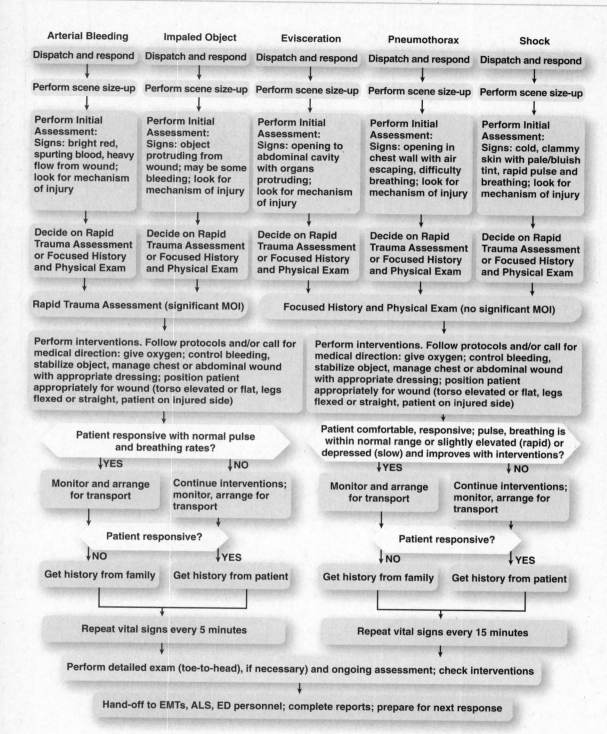

Arterial Bleeding	Impaled Object	Evisceration	Pneumothorax	Shock

Dispatch and respond → **Perform scene size-up**

Arterial Bleeding — Perform Initial Assessment: Signs: bright red, spurting blood, heavy flow from wound; look for mechanism of injury

Impaled Object — Perform Initial Assessment: Signs: object protruding from wound; may be some bleeding; look for mechanism of injury

Evisceration — Perform Initial Assessment: Signs: opening to abdominal cavity with organs protruding; look for mechanism of injury

Pneumothorax — Perform Initial Assessment: Signs: opening in chest wall with air escaping, difficulty breathing; look for mechanism of injury

Shock — Perform Initial Assessment: Signs: cold, clammy skin with pale/bluish tint, rapid pulse and breathing; look for mechanism of injury

Decide on Rapid Trauma Assessment or Focused History and Physical Exam

Rapid Trauma Assessment (significant MOI)

Focused History and Physical Exam (no significant MOI)

Perform interventions. Follow protocols and/or call for medical direction: give oxygen; control bleeding, stabilize object, manage chest or abdominal wound with appropriate dressing; position patient appropriately for wound (torso elevated or flat, legs flexed or straight, patient on injured side)

Patient responsive with normal pulse and breathing rates?
- ↓YES — **Monitor and arrange for transport**
- ↓NO — **Continue interventions; monitor, arrange for transport**

Patient responsive?
- ↓NO — **Get history from family**
- ↓YES — **Get history from patient**

Repeat vital signs every 5 minutes

Patient comfortable, responsive; pulse, breathing is within normal range or slightly elevated (rapid) or depressed (slow) and improves with interventions?
- ↓YES — **Monitor and arrange for transport**
- ↓NO — **Continue interventions; monitor, arrange for transport**

Patient responsive?
- ↓NO — **Get history from family**
- ↓YES — **Get history from patient**

Repeat vital signs every 15 minutes

Perform detailed exam (toe-to-head), if necessary) and ongoing assessment; check interventions

Hand-off to EMTs, ALS, ED personnel; complete reports; prepare for next response

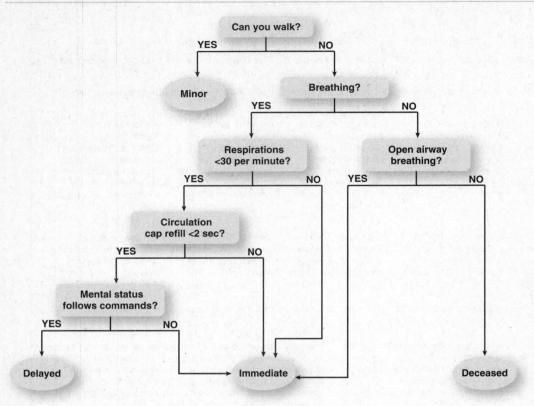

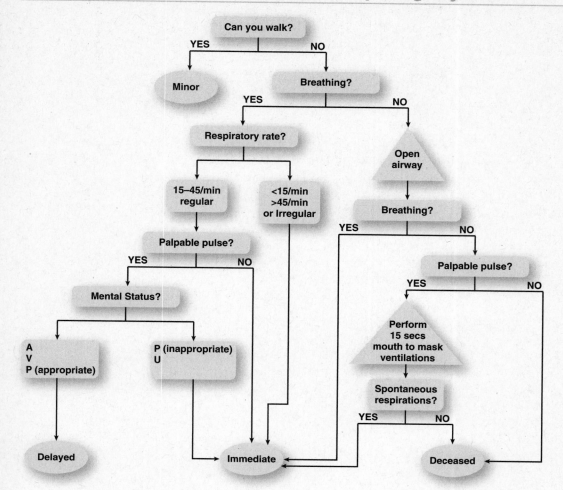

© 2009 by Pearson Education, Inc. *First Responder*, Eighth Edition, Bergeron et al.

Answer Key

The following answers are for the Exercises section in each workbook chapter, the Module Reviews, Appendices, and the Posttest. Note that page references where answers can be found in the textbook are provided in parentheses.

CHAPTER 1: INTRODUCTION TO EMS SYSTEMS

EXERCISES

1. (p. 4)

2. (p. 7)

3. law enforcement officers, members of the fire service, Medical Emergency Response Teams, Life Guards, private citizens (p. 11)

4. personal safety (p. 10)

5. A) safely gain access to the patient; B) find out what is wrong with the patient and provide emergency care; C) lift or move the patient only when required and do so without causing additional injury; D) transfer the patient and patient information to more highly trained personnel when they arrive at the scene; E) maintain strict confidentiality regarding patient information; F) act as an advocate for the patient (pp. 12–13)

6. (pp. 14–15)

7. Emergency Medical Responder, EMT, Advanced EMT, Paramedic (p. 7)

8. (pp. 12–13)

CHAPTER 2: LEGAL AND ETHICAL ISSUES

EXERCISES

1. (p. 22)

2. (pp. 23–24)

3. (pp. 24–25)

4. A) C; B) A; C) B; D) D (pp. 25–26)

5. (pp. 27–28)

6. In many states it is usually when an EMR is on duty or once they have begun care. (p. 28)

7. Duty, Breach of Duty, Damages, Causation (p. 28)

© 2009 by Pearson Education, Inc. *First Responder*, Eighth Edition, Bergeron et al.

8. (p. 29)

9. (pp. 29–30)

10. (pp. 30–32)

11. (p. 32)

12. (p. 32)

13. (p. 33)

14. (pp. 33–34)

CHAPTER 3: WELL-BEING OF THE EMERGENCY MEDICAL RESPONDER

EXERCISES

1. A) recognize the patient's needs; B) be tolerant of angry reactions from the patients or family members; C) listen empathetically; D) do not give false hope or reassurance; E) offer comfort (p. 40)

2. (p. 43)

3. Any three: develop healthful and positive dietary habits; exercise; devote time to relaxing; change work environments or shifts; seek professional help (pp. 43–45)

4. (p. 46)

5. (p. 46)

6. gloves—any patient contact; face masks—blood or fluid spatter, any time airborne pathogens are present; eye protection—any time splashing is possible; gowns—arterial bleeding, childbirth, or multiple injuries with heavy bleeding (p. 48)

7. (pp. 53–54)

8. A) B; B) C; C) A (pp. 54–55)

CHAPTER 4: THE HUMAN BODY

EXERCISES

1. Figure 4.1 (p. 60)

2. shoulder joint, arm, elbow, forearm, wrist, hand (p. 63)

3. Figure 4.4 (p. 64)

4. right upper quadrant—liver, gall bladder, or part of the large intestine; left upper quadrant—stomach, spleen, or part of the large intestine; right lower quadrant—appendix, part of the urinary bladder, or part of the large intestine; left lower quadrant—part of the large intestine or part of the urinary bladder (p. 65)

5. circulatory system—moves blood, carries oxygen and nutrients to the cells, and removes carbon dioxide and wastes; respiratory system—exchanges air to bring in oxygen and expel carbon dioxide; digestive system—digests and absorbs foods and removes certain wastes; urinary system—removes chemical wastes from the blood and helps to balance water and salt levels of the blood; reproductive system—produces all structures and hormones necessary for

© 2009 by Pearson Education, Inc. *First Responder*, Eighth Edition, Bergeron et al.

sexual reproduction; nervous system—controls movement, interprets sensations, regulates body activities, generates memory and thought; endocrine system—produces hormones that regulate most body activities and functions; musculoskeletal system—protects and supports the body and permits body movement; special senses—provides sight, hearing, taste, smell, and the sensations of hot, cold, pain, and tactile responses (pp. 65–67)

6. Figures 4.6 (p. 68)

7. Figure 4.8 (p. 68)

8. Figure 4.9 (p. 69)

9. Figure 4.10 (p. 69)

CHAPTER 5: LIFTING, MOVING, AND POSITIONING PATIENTS

EXERCISES

1. (p. 85)

2. responsive patient, initial assessment completed, pulse and breathing rates stable and within normal ranges, no serious bleeding, no neck or spinal injuries, all suspected fractures and extremity injuries properly immobilized (p. 88)

3. A) E; B) E; C) N; D) E; E) N (pp. 86–94)

4. any four: shoulder, clothes, foot, blanket, incline, firefighter's (p. 87)

5. one-rescuer assist (p. 89)

6. length, or long axis, to keep the spine in alignment (p. 86)

7. (pp. 90–91)

8. (pp. 98–103)

MODULE 1 REVIEW

1.	B (p. 4)	14.	C (p. 26)
2.	C (p. 8)	15.	A (p. 26)
3.	C (p. 10)	16.	C (p. 27)
4.	D (pp. 12–13)	17.	C (p. 29)
5.	D (p. 14)	18.	C (p. 29)
6.	B (p. 45)	19.	A (pp. 29–30)
7.	D (p. 46)	20.	D (p. 31)
8.	B (p. 47)	21.	D (p. 60)
9.	D (p. 51)	22.	A (p. 61)
10.	D (p. 51)	23.	C (p. 61)
11.	A (p. 52)	24.	B (p. 61)
12.	B (p. 22)	25.	A (p. 64)
13.	C (pp. 24–25)	26.	D (p. 65)

27. B (p. 63)
28. A (p. 65)
29. Scan 4–1 (p. 70)
30. C (p. 86)
31. D (p. 89)

32. D (p. 88)
33. B (p. 90)
34. A (pp. 86–92)
35. C (p. 98)

CHAPTER 6: AIRWAY MANAGEMENT

EXERCISES

1. (p. 115)

2. (pp. 115–116)

3. (p. 119)

4. Look for . . . the even and effortless rise and fall of the chest.

   Listen for . . . air entering and leaving. Sounds should be quiet.

   Feel for . . . air moving in and out of the mouth and nose.

   Observe . . . skin color; it should not be pale, or bluish. (p. 119)

5. Figure 6.4 (p. 118)

6. (p. 119)

   - Little or no chest rise and fall
   - Uneven chest rise and fall
   - No air exchange heard or felt at nose or mouth
   - Noisy breathing
   - Irregular, rapid, or slow breathing
   - Shallow, deep, or labored breathing
   - Pale or bluish skin
   - Difficulty breathing
   - Flared nostrils
   - Breathing that uses accessory muscles
   - Patient sitting or leaning forward in the tripod position.

7. (pp. 120–121)

8. (pp. 121–122)

9. A) reduces the effort required to keep the patient's airway open; B) prevents contact with the patient's mouth, nose, blood, body fluids (pp. 122–123)

10. A) Open airway; B) Check breathing; C) Provide rescue breaths; D) Watch for chest rise and fall (pp. 123–124)

11. one, 5–6 seconds (p. 124)

12. (p. 124)

13. (p. 128)

14. complete airway obstruction (p. 131)

15. A) unable to speak or cough; B) will grasp neck and open mouth widely as a distress sign for choking (p. 131)

16. A) tongue in the back of the throat; B) tissue damage from trauma; C) foreign object in the throat; D) tissue swelling (Figure 6.12, p. 130)

17. A) D; B) B; C) A; D) C (p. 131)
18. five (p. 134)
19. (pp. 134–135)
20. inward, upward (p. 132)
21. nipples (p. 137)
22. chest (p. 136)
23. (p. 137)
24. A) confirm complete obstruction; B) perform up to five manual (abdominal or chest) thrusts; C) repeat manual thrusts until the airway is cleared or the patient becomes unresponsive (pp. 132–134)
25. (p. 134)
26. adequate ventilations (p. 134)
27. oropharyngeal, nasopharyngeal (p. 138)
28. mouth, throat, unresponsive (p. 138)
29. (pp. 139–142)
30. (pp. 146–147)

MODULE 2 REVIEW

1. C (p. 115)
2. D (p. 117)
3. C (p. 117)
4. D (p. 121)
5. C (p. 122)
6. C (pp. 123–124)
7. A (p. 124)
8. B (p. 124)
9. A (p. 124)
10. B (p. 128)
11. A (p. 130)
12. B (p. 130)
13. C (p. 131)
14. A (p. 131)
15. B (p. 134)
16. D (p. 137)
17. D (p. 134)
18. B (p. 135)
19. B (p. 136)
20. C (p. 138)
21. A (p. 138)
22. B (p. 139)
23. C (pp. 139–140)
24. D (p. 141)
25. C (p. 146)

CHAPTER 7: ASSESSMENT OF THE PATIENT

EXERCISES

1. Assessment-based care does not require that a specific cause or problem be defined. Instead, general categories can be used to select care procedures (in most cases). (p. 157)
2. A) ensure your own safety; B) make the scene safe for the patient; C) find out if the patient is responsive; D) form a general impression of the patient (pp. 158–159)

© 2009 by Pearson Education, Inc. *First Responder*, Eighth Edition, Bergeron et al.

3. A) scene size-up; B) initial assessment; C) focused history and physical exam; D) detailed physical exam; E) ongoing assessment (p. 167)

4. First: identify and provide for life-threatening problems.
   Second: identify other injuries or medical problems and provide care.
   Third: monitor the patient for changing conditions. (p. 163)

5. A) scene safety; B) mechanism of injury or nature of illness; C) number of patients; D) need for additional resources; E) consider need for spinal precautions (p. 165)

6. (p. 164)

7. (p. 168)

8. A) form a general impression of the patient; B) assess the patient's mental status; C) assess the patient's airway; D) assess the patient's breathing; E) assess the patient's circulation (pulse and bleeding); F) make a decision on the priority of the patient for transport (pp. 168–170)

9. Airway (ensure an open airway); Breathing (maintain airway/rescue breathing); Circulation (chest compressions/control bleeding) (p. 168)

10. (p. 168)

11. A—alert; V—responsive to verbal stimuli; P—responsive to painful stimuli; U—unresponsive (pp. 170, 172)

12. LOOK for: chest movement associated with breathing.
    LISTEN for: the movement of air at the patient's mouth and nose.
    FEEL for: air being exhaled. (p. 172)

13. carotid pulse (p. 174)

14. (pp. 174–175)

15. (p. 175)

16. (p. 175)

17. to detect and care for the patient's specific injuries or medical problems (p. 176)

18. A) Focused trauma assessment; B) Rapid trauma assessment; C) Rapid medical assessment; D) Focused medical assessment (pp. 176–177)

19. allergies—penicillin, etc.; medications—aspirin, etc.; past medical history—heart attack, etc.; last oral intake—dinner; events leading up to the event—at rest (p. 183)

20. A) What is the patient's name?

    B) What happened?

    C) Did you see anything else?

    D) Did the patient complain of anything?

    E) Did the patient have any known illness or problem?

    F) Do you know if the patient was taking any medications? (pp. 183–184)

21. When the problem that you find could be life threatening to the patient. (p. 177)

22. (p. 166)

23. Deformities, Contusions, Abrasions, Punctures/Penetrations, Burns, Tenderness, Lacerations, Swelling (p. 191)

24. Bleeding, Pain, Deformities, Open wounds, Crepitus (p. 191)

25. rhythm, strength (p. 185)

26. (p. 187)

27. infant—120 to 160; child/1–5 years—80 to 140; child/5–12 years—70 to 110; adult—60 to 100 (p. 186)

28. adult—12 to 20; child/6–10 years—15 to 30; child/1–5 years—20 to 30; infant—30 to 50 (p. 188)

29. A) 2   I) 12   P) 19
    B) 9   J) 13   Q) 6
    C) 20   K) 14   R) 5
    D) 7   L) 11   S) 4
    E) 18   M) 10   T) 17
    F) 3   N) 15   U) 1
    G) 16   O) 8   V) 22
    H) 21   (pp. 192–196)

30. A) touch each toe; B) have patient push foot against your hand; C) pinch the top of the foot; D) check capillary refill time (p. 195)

31. Pinch the back of each hand. (p. 196)

32. (p. 198)

33. (pp. 198–199)

34. (pp. 196–197)

MODULE 3 REVIEW

1. B (p. 157)
2. A (p. 181)
3. C (pp. 172–175)
4. A (p. 168)
5. D (p. 172)
6. A (p. 174)
7. A (p. 174)
8. C (p. 157)
9. B (p. 157)
10. B (p. 177)
11. C (p. 177)
12. D (p. 177)
13. B (p. 182)
14. C (p. 183)
15. C (p. 183)
16. B (p. 185)
17. B (p. 186)
18. B (p. 187)
19. C (p. 188)
20. A (p. 188)
21. D (p. 191)
22. B (p. 197)
23. A (p. 193)
24. C (p. 199)
25. A (p. 199)

CHAPTER 8: RESUSCITATION AND USE OF THE AED

EXERCISES

1. early access to EMS; early CPR; early defibrillation; early advanced cardiac life support (ACLS) (pp. 206–207)

2. A) patient is unresponsive; B) patient is not breathing; C) patient does not have a pulse (p. 208)

3. airway, breathing, circulation (p. 208)

4. When breathing and heartbeat stop (p. 115)

5. four, six (p. 207)

6. biological death; the brain (p. 208)

7. (pp. 208–209)

8. (p. 216)

9. A) form a general impression; B) assess responsiveness; C) assess airway; D) assess breathing; E) assess circulation; F) position the patient and begin CPR (p. 210)

10. (pp. 213–214)

11. A) deliver each breath over 1 second; B) provide two slow breaths after every thirty compressions; C) do not overventilate the patient; D) establish a regular pattern of breathing for yourself (p. 214)

12. 100, 30 (p. 215)

13. Line 3: head, lift

    Line 4: feel

    Line 5: two

    Line 6: clear

    Line 7: carotid

    Line 10: 30

    Line 11: two

    Line 12: 2 minutes or 5 cycles

    Line 13: first (pp. 216–219)

14. Line 7: carotid, brachial, apical

    Line 8: 30 (pp. 220–226)

15. A) patient is placed on a hard, flat surface; B) the airway is opened with the correct technique; C) the mouth and nose are sealed with a barrier; D) the nostrils are pinched shut; E) the hands are placed over the proper compression site; F) the compressions are performed to the proper depth and pressure is relaxed to allow the heart to fill; G) the correct rates and ratios are used; H) the necessary interruptions are limited to 3-to-5-second pulse and breathing checks and 15-to-30-second patient moves. (p. 227)

16. (p. 227)

17. A) spontaneous circulation begins; B) spontaneous breathing and circulation begin; C) an equally or higher trained member of the EMS system takes over for you; D) you turn over responsibility to a physician; E) you are exhausted. (p. 231)

18. Adult: Heels of two hands, 1.5 to 2 inches, approximately 100 per minute, 30:2 Child: Heel of one hand, 1/2 to 1/3 the depth of the chest, approximately 100 per minute, 30:2 Infant: Two or three fingers, . 1/2 to 1/3 the depth of the chest, at least 100 per minute, 30:2 (p. 228)

19. (p. 232)

20. (pp. 232–233)

21. (pp. 235–236)

22. (pp. 237–238) *Note:* Make certain that you follow local protocols.

23. Stop CPR. (p. 237)

24. Check breathing and pulse. (p. 238)

25. pads, cables (p. 239)

26. (p. 237)

MODULE 4 REVIEW

1.	C (p. 208)	12.	D (p. 224)
2.	C (p. 208)	13.	B (p. 225)
3.	C (p. 210)	14.	D (p. 225)
4.	D (p. 214)	15.	D (p. 226)
5.	C (p. 213)	16.	D (p. 227)
6.	B (p. 214)	17.	A (p. 232)
7.	C (p. 216)	18.	C (p. 236)
8.	B (p. 213)	19.	C (p. 238)
9.	D (p. 215)	20.	A (p. 239)
10.	B (p. 223)	21.	B (p. 239)
11.	D (p. 216)	22.	D (p. 222)

© 2009 by Pearson Education, Inc. *First Responder*, Eighth Edition, Bergeron et al.

CHAPTER 9: CARING FOR MEDICAL EMERGENCIES

EXERCISES

1. signs are what you observe; symptoms are what the patient tells you about his condition (p. 249)

2. (p. 249)

3. (p. 249)

4. A) complete a scene size-up; B) complete an initial assessment; C) complete an appropriate history and physical exam; D) complete ongoing assessments (as appropriate); E) comfort and reassure the patient while awaiting additional EMS resources (p. 249)

5. (p. 252)

6. "Your pain could be a lot of things, but let's not take any chances." (p. 258)

7. (pp. 252, 254–255)

8. volume of respirations, how easy (p. 259)

9. (p. 259)

10. A) C; B) D; C) A; D) B; E) E (pp. 264, 267–268, 282)

11. No; objects placed in a patient's mouth could break off and obstruct the airway. (p. 268)

12. A) ingestion; B) inhalation; C) absorption; D) injection. Examples given will vary. (p. 274)

13. Check with your instructor on local policy. (p. 276)

14. coughing, shortness of breath; evidence of possible sources: stoves, charcoal, auto exhaust, industrial solvents, and spray cans (p. 278)

15. flooding, water (p. 280)

16. skin: itchy, rash, swelling; breathing: difficulty breathing, throat swelling; pulse: rapid, very weak, or not detected; face: lips turn blue, tongue and face may swell; mental status: restlessness, followed by lowered level of consciousness (p. 282)

17. (pp. 280–283)

18. (pp. 284–285)

19. Because the body's temperature-regulating mechanism fails and the body is unable to rid itself of excess heat, the body temperature can go as high as 105°. (p. 286)

20. chill (p. 286)

21. hypothermia (p. 286)

22. DO: (Any two)

Perform scene size-up.

Make sure someone alerts dispatch.

Perform an initial assessment.

Remove patient from cold environment.

Protect patient from further heat loss.

Remove wet clothing and place blanket over patient.

Handle patient gently.

Comfort and reassure patient while awaiting additional EMS.

Monitor vital signs.

DO NOT:

Allow the patient to walk or exert himself.

Give the patient anything to eat or drink. (p. 287)

23. frostbite; fingers, toes, ears, face, nose (p. 288)

24. These substances may constrict blood vessels and worsen the condition. (p. 287)

25. A) situational stress; B) mind-altering substances; C) psychiatric problems; D) psychological crises (p. 290)

26. (pp. 291–292)

27. (p. 292)

28. (p. 296)

CHAPTER 10: CARING FOR BLEEDING, SHOCK, AND SOFT-TISSUE INJURIES

EXERCISES

1. A) carry oxygen and carbon dioxide; B) carry food to the tissues; C) carry waste from the tissues to the organs of excretion; D) carry hormones, water, salts, and other compounds needed to keep the body's functions in balance; E) protect against disease-causing organisms. (p. 306)

2. (pp. 307–308, 320)

3. artery—function: carries blood away from the heart; color and flow: bright red and spurting; vein—function: returns blood to the heart; color and flow: dark red and steady flow; capillary—function: where oxygen, nutrient, and waste exchange takes place; color and flow: red (less bright than arterial) and oozing. (pp. 307–308)

4. arterial bleeding is generally most severe because the pressure is greater inside these vessels (p. 308)

5. A) direct pressure; B) elevation; C) pressure points; D) tourniquet (p. 310)

6. direct pressure, elevation, pressure point; tourniquet (pp. 309–311)

7. elevation (p. 313)

8. A) control bleeding; B) use sterile or clean materials; C) cover the entire wound; D) do not remove dressings (p. 319)

9. A) do not bandage too tightly; B) do not bandage too loosely; C) do not leave loose ends; D) do not cover fingers and toes; E) bandage from the bottom of a limb to the top (pp. 319–320)

10. (p. 322)

11. shock (p. 322)

12. (pp. 322–323)

13. A) Make certain that someone alerts the EMS dispatcher.

    B) Perform scene size-up, including BSI.

    C) Perform initial assessment.

    D) Keep the patient in the proper position and lying still.

    E) Loosen restrictive clothing and provide care for shock.

    F) Be alert in case the patient starts to vomit.

    G) Do not give the patient anything by mouth.

    H) Apply pressure dressings if internal bleeding is in an extremity.

    I) Reassure patient and keep patient calm.

    J) Report the possibility of internal bleeding to more highly trained EMS professionals. (p. 324)

14. (p. 325)

15. decrease in blood pressure, increase in heart rate, pale skin (pp. 323, 327–328)

16. (p. 327)

17. (p. 327)

18. (pp. 329–330)

© 2009 by Pearson Education, Inc. *First Responder,* Eighth Edition, Bergeron et al.

19. A closed wound is an internal injury in which the skin is not broken. In an open wound, the skin is opened. (p. 332)

20. A) E; B) A; C) H; D) D; E) B; F) G; G) F; H) C (pp. 332–334)

21. A) Expose the wound.

   B)   Clear the wound surface.

   C)   Control bleeding.

   D)   Prevent further contamination.

   E)   Keep the patient lying still.

   F)   Reassure the patient.

   G)   Care for shock. (pp. 335–337)

22. An object through the cheek may be blocking the patient's airway or may break loose and fall into the airway. (p. 342)

23. occlusive dressing. This will prevent air from being sucked back into the chest through the wound. (p. 351)

24. (p. 355)

25. (p. 356)

26. (p. 356)

27. A)   Perform an initial assessment.

   B)   For major burns, do not flush with water, remove smoldering clothing and jewelry, continue to monitor airway.

   C)   Do not use ointment, lotion, or antiseptic.

   D)   Do not break blisters.

   E)   Give special care to the eyes.

   F)   Give special care to the fingers and toes.

   G)   Continue to ensure a clear and open airway, remembering that burns to the face or exposure to smoke or hot gases may cause severe airway problems. (pp. 357–358)

28. 20 (p. 360)

CHAPTER 11: CARING FOR MUSCLE AND BONE INJURIES

EXERCISES

1. A) support; B) movement; C) protection; D) blood cell production (pp. 369–370)

2. skull, spinal column, sternum, ribs (p. 370)

3. A)   Shoulder blade (scapula)

   B)   Collarbone (clavicle)

   C)   Arm bone (humerus)

   D)   Lateral forearm bone (radius)

   E)   Medial forearm bone (ulna)

   F)   Thigh bone (femur)

G) Kneecap (patella)

H) Medial lower leg bone (tibia)

I) Lateral lower leg bone (fibula) (pp. 371–373)

4. A) indirect; B) direct; C) twisting (p. 374)

5. discoloration, exposed bone ends, inability to move (pp. 377–378)

6. (p. 379)

7. A) low; B) high; C) medium; D) medium; E) high; F) low; G) high (pp. 379–380)

8. A) Carefully expose the injury site.

B) Immobilize the extremity.

C) Apply a cold pack.

D) Give oxygen per local protocols.

E) Cover the patient to maintain body temperature. (pp. 380–381)

F) immobilizing, stabilizing, splint (pp. 381–382)

9. soft and rigid (pp. 386, 388)

10. (pp. 382–384)

11. A) A; B) E; C) A; D) E; E) B (p. 384)

12. ankle—ankle hitch

knee—rigid splint most effective, but can use soft splint

thigh—traction splint

hip—blanket roll, long rigid splint (pp. 399–404)

13. (p. 409)

14. A) Provide resuscitative measures.

B) Control bleeding.

C) Dress and bandage open wounds and stabilize penetrating objects.

D) Monitor and record all vital signs.

E) Be prepared for vomiting. (p. 411)

15. A) cervical vertebrae; B) thoracic vertebrae; C) lumbar vertebrae; D) sacral vertebrae; E) coccygeal vertebrae (fused) (p. 76)

16. A) S; B) F; C) S; D) F; E) B; F) S; G) F (pp. 413–414, 425–426)

17. A) Make certain the airway is open, assist ventilations, or perform CPR as needed.

B) Attempt to control serious bleeding.

C) Always assume that an unresponsive trauma patient has spinal injuries.

D) Do not attempt to splint fractures if there are indications of spinal injuries until you have appropriate help.

E) Never move a patient unless it is to control life-threatening bleeding or perform CPR.

F) Keep the patient still. Tell her not to move.

G) Continuously monitor patients with possible spinal injuries. (p. 417)

© 2009 by Pearson Education, Inc. *First Responder*, Eighth Edition, Bergeron et al.

18. (p. 418)

19.
  A) Locate the flail segment.

  B) Apply a bulky dressing.

  C) Use large strips of tape to hold in place.

  D) Provide oxygen per protocols.

  E) Monitor the patient to assure adequate breathing. (pp. 426–427)

CHAPTER 12: CARING FOR THE GERIATRIC PATIENT

EXERCISES

1. Many elderly patients have multiple illnesses at any given time. This means that they will be presenting with many different signs and symptoms, making it difficult for the EMR to prioritize or define what the primary complaint is. (p. 434)

2. multiple illnesses, multiple medications, decreased mobility, decreased hearing and sight, difficulty communicating, incontinence, altered mental status (pp. 434-436)

3. respiratory, cardiac, nervous, musculoskeletal, skin (pp. 437–440)

4. difficulty hearing, multiple layers of clothing, multiple illnesses (pp. 434, 441)

5. COPD, Alzheimer's, Parkinson's, congestive heart failure, high blood pressure, stroke (pp. 441-442)

MODULE 5 REVIEW

1.	C (p. 251)		**18.**	A (p. 330)
2.	C (p. 265)		**19.**	A (p. 342)
3.	A (pp. 254–255)		**20.**	C (p. 346)
4.	C (p. 258)		**21.**	D (p. 347)
5.	D (p. 257)		**22.**	D (pp. 349–350)
6.	C (p. 268)		**23.**	C (p. 356)
7.	A (p. 277)		**24.**	B (pp. 357–358)
8.	C (p. 281)		**25.**	B (p. 360)
9.	A (p. 284)		**26.**	D (p. 360)
10.	C (p. 288)		**27.**	D (p. 419)
11.	B (p. 289)		**28.**	A (p. 398)
12.	C (p. 306)		**29.**	C (p. 404)
13.	D (p. 306)		**30.**	B (p. 397)
14.	A (p. 306)		**31.**	D (p. 396)
15.	B (p. 307)		**32.**	C (p. 400)
16.	D (p. 309)		**33.**	B (p. 401)
17.	B (pp. 322–323)		**34.**	C (p. 418)

35.	B (p. 409)	43.	B (p. 417)
36.	A (p. 409)	44.	D (p. 424)
37.	A (p. 411)	45.	B (p. 424)
38.	C (p. 411)	46.	B (p. 440)
39.	D (p. 411)	47.	C (p. 437)
40.	A (p. 411)	48.	A (p. 437)
41.	C (p. 414)	49.	D (p. 436)
42.	B (p. 419)	50.	A (p. 434)

CHAPTER 13: CHILDBIRTH

EXERCISES

1. The first stage begins when contractions begin and ends with the full dilation of the cervix (10 centimeters). The second stage begins with full dilation of the cervix and ends with the delivery of the baby. The third stage begins following delivery of the baby and ends with delivery of the placenta. (p. 452)

2. (pp. 452–453)

3. A) the mother says she feels the baby trying to be born; B) contractions are less than two minutes apart; C) the mother is straining, crying out, complaining about having to go to the bathroom. (p. 456)

4. See Figure 13.1. (p. 451)

5. A)   What is patient's name, age, and expected due date?

   B)   Has the patient been under a doctor's care?

   C)   Is this her first pregnancy?

   D)   Has she discharged any watery or bloody mucus?

   E)   How long has she been having labor pains?

   F)   Has her water broken and when?

   G)   Does she feel strain in her abdomen or pelvis?

   H)   Does she have any significant medical information (e.g., seizures, diabetes)? (p. 455)

6. A)   Control the scene.

   B)   Position the mother.

   C)   Feel the abdomen for contractions.

   D)   Prepare the mother for examination.

   E)   Check for crowning.

   F)   Do not attempt any vaginal or internal examination. (pp. 456–457)

7. A) latex or vinyl gloves; B) gown; C) eye protection; D) face shields (p. 454)

8. Crowning; place one hand below the baby's head as it delivers. Spread your fingers evenly around the head to support it, but avoid pressing on the soft spots. Apply a slight pressure on the head to control the delivery speed. (pp. 451, 460)

9. A)   Clear the baby's airway.

   B)   Make certain the baby is breathing.

   C)   Perform a quick assessment.

© 2009 by Pearson Education, Inc. *First Responder*, Eighth Edition, Bergeron et al.

D) Clamp or tie off the cord.

E) Keep the baby warm.

F) If tape is available, write the mother's last name and delivery time on a piece of tape. Loop it around the baby's wrist. (pp. 461–463)

10. Vigorously but gently rub the baby's back. Snap one of your index fingers against the soles of the baby's feet. However, do not hold the baby up by the feet and slap its bottom. (pp. 462)

11. (p. 464)

12. Try to position a basin or container at the vaginal opening so the afterbirth will deliver into it. After collecting it, wrap the container in a towel, newspaper, or plastic wrap. If no container is available, allow the afterbirth to deliver into a towel or newspaper. It should be saved so that it may be examined by a physician. (p. 467)

13. (pp. 467–468)

14. A) B; B) A; C) E; D) C; E) D (pp. 469–473)

15. A) Take an initial set of vital signs.

B) Provide care for shock and place patient on her side.

C) Place a sanitary pad over the opening to the vagina. Do not place anything into the vagina.

D) Save all blood-soaked pads and any tissues that are passed.

E) Provide emotional support.

F) Arrange for transport immediately. (p. 470)

16. Breech birth:

Support the baby as it emerges.

If baby's head does not deliver within 3 minutes, create an airway.

Maintain the airway.

Allow 3 minutes for delivery.

Give a high concentration of oxygen. (pp. 471–472)

Prolapsed cord:

Do not try to push the cord back into the birth canal.

Place the mother in a knee-chest position.

Place wet dressings over the cord; wrap it in a towel to keep it warm.

Give the mother a high concentration of oxygen. (p. 473)

Premature birth:

Dry the baby and keep him warm.

Cover his head and transfer him to a warm environment.

If necessary, resuscitate using mouth-to-mask or mouth-to-mouth-and-nose.

Clear secretions from his mouth and nose before ventilating. (pp. 473–474)

17. (pp. 475–476)

18. (p. 477)

CHAPTER 14: CARING FOR INFANTS AND CHILDREN

EXERCISES

1. (p. 489)

Newborn	birth to 1 year
Toddler	1 to 3 years
Preschool	3 to 6 years old
School Age	6 to 12 years old
Adolescent	12 to 18 years old

2. larger; heavier (p. 492)

3. Figure 14.2 (p. 485)

4. You may unintentionally force and wedge the obstruction farther into the narrow pharynx and trachea. (pp. 137 and 497)

5. adolescent: 12 to 20

   child: 15 to 30

   infant: 25 to 50

   neonate: 40 to 60 (p. 494)

6. less than 2 (p. 493)

7. 3 to 5 (p. 498)

8. A) Is the child alert, struggling to breathe, crying, quiet, or listless?

   B) Is the skin pale, bluish, or flushed?

   C) How is the child interacting with the environment?

   D) What is the child's body position? (pp. 495–496)

9. The child has an adequate airway, breathing, and circulation. (p. 496)

10. Any four:

    gives a poor general impression

    is unresponsive or listless

    has an airway problem

    is in respiratory arrest, or has inadequate breathing or respiratory distress

    has a possibility of developing shock

    has uncontrolled bleeding (p. 496)

11. The head-to-toe assessment that you perform on adults is usually reversed and performed in toe-to-head order. (p. 485)

12. Any five: wheezing, an effort to exhale, breathing that is faster or slower than normal, child in the tripod position, drooling, nasal flaring, cyanosis, capillary refill of more than 2 seconds, altered mental status (p. 502)

13. Loud wheezing and breath sounds, becoming less audible as the attack worsens; shortness of breath; obvious respiratory distress with easy inhalation and forced expiration; cough; faster

than normal breathing; increased heart rate, faster and weaker pulse; sleepiness or slowed response; skin color changes, often to the blue or gray, particularly around the lips and eyes. In some cases, bronchial spasms may appear rapidly, and the airways will narrow quickly; if so be prepared for the swift buildup of fluids or mucus. (p. 502)

14. Any three: high fever, epilepsy, infections, poisoning, hypoglycemia, head injury, low oxygen (p. 503)

15. A) Maintain an open airway and insert nothing into the mouth.

B) Look for evidence of injury.

C) If you do not suspect injury, position the child on his side.

D) Be alert for vomiting.

E) Provide oxygen or assisted ventilations with supplemental oxygen.

F) Monitor breathing and altered mental status. (p. 504)

16. Any three: hypoglycemia, poisoning, infection, head injury, decreased oxygen levels, shock, period after seizure (p. 504)

17. hypoperfusion (children can compensate for a long time but compensating mechanisms can fail suddenly) (pp. 504–505)

18. Explain that the cause of SIDS is unknown; however, it is known that the cause of death is not the fault of the parents. Many parents will still wonder if there was something else they could have done. Let them know that there is no reason for guilt, only for sorrow. (p. 506)

19. fever, long bouts of diarrhea and vomiting, and little fluid intake, or rapid temperature rise with or without seizure (p. 507)

20. (p. 485)

21. head; the surface area of the child's head is proportionately larger than the rest of the body; the large head radiates and loses heat when it is uncovered. (p. 508)

22. Any three:

Do undress the child but do not allow him to be chilled.

Do cover the child with a towel soaked in tepid water.

Do place damp, cold cloths on the fevered child's head.

Do give sips of cool water or let the child suck on a cloth filled with chipped ice.

Do transport any child who has a seizure. (pp. 507–508)

23. A) never submerge the child in cold water

B) never use rubbing alcohol for cooling (p. 508)

24. A) psychological (emotional) abuse; B) neglect; C) physical abuse; D) sexual abuse (p. 518)

25. Arrange for transportation and report suspicions to the EMTs providing transport, the hospital staff, or the appropriate law enforcement agency. (p. 518)

MODULE 6 REVIEW

1. D (p. 451)
2. C (p. 451)
3. B (p. 452)
4. C (p. 452)
5. B (p. 452)
6. C (p. 452)

7. C (p. 455)
8. D (p. 457)
9. C (p. 460)
10. C (p. 460)
11. B (p. 460)
12. B (p. 460)
13. A (p. 462)
14. C (p. 462)
15. C (p. 461)
16. A (p. 461)
17. B (p. 467)
18. B (p. 471)
19. A (p. 472)
20. C (pp. 473–474)
21. C (p. 485)
22. B (p. 489)
23. D (p. 492)

24. C (p. 492)
25. D (p. 494)
26. A (p. 496)
27. B (p. 497)
28. A (p. 496)
29. B (p. 498)
30. D (p. 501)
31. B (p. 502)
32. B (p. 504)
33. C (p. 505)
34. A (p. 506)
35. C (p. 507)
36. B (p. 508)
37. D (p. 508)
38. A (p. 510)
39. C (p. 514)
40. B (p. 518)

© 2009 by Pearson Education, Inc. *First Responder*, Eighth Edition, Bergeron et al.

CHAPTER 15: EMS OPERATIONS

EXERCISES

1. Follow standard operating guidelines; limit your actions to your training level; use the proper equipment and the required number of trained persons for any task. (p. 530)

2. A) Evaluate the scene.

   B) Wear proper protective gear.

   C) Do only what you have been trained to do.

   D) Call the dispatcher for the appropriate assistance. (p. 530)

3. A) Preparation—proper training, tools, and equipment

   B) Dispatch—be familiar with dispatch procedures and note information dispatch gives about the call.

   C) En route to the scene—fasten seat belts, have PPE ready, contact dispatch.

   D) Arrival at the scene—approach cautiously, notify dispatch, don PPE.

   E) Transferring patients—assist in preparing and moving patients for transport.

   F). After the emergency—clean and disinfect equipment, complete paperwork, notify dispatch. (pp. 531–533)

4. fire; leaking fuel or gases; unstable vehicles; downed electrical wires (p. 534)

5. B) a window; C) doors; D) the metal (p. 537)

6. A) Stabilize it with tires, blocks, lumber, and so on.

B)   Use rope to tie the vehicle to secure objects.

C)   Gain access to the occupants through the rear window.

D)   If you open a door, tie it securely open. (pp. 540–541)

7.   (pp. 541–542)

8.   (p. 543)

9.   (pp. 543–544)

10.   (pp. 544–545)

11.   (p. 545)

12.   (p. 546)

13.   protect oneself; hot zone; cold zone (p. 547)

14.   danger; safe (p. 547)

15.   (pp. 547–548)

16.   (p. 549)

CHAPTER 16: MULTIPLE-CASUALTY INCIDENTS, TRIAGE, AND THE INCIDENT MANAGEMENT SYSTEM

EXERCISES

1.   (p. 558)

2.   A)   respirations greater than or less than 30 per minute

   B)   perfusion; capillary refill time is either greater than or less than 2 seconds

   C)   mental status; can patient follow simple commands? (p. 559)

3.   (pp. 558–560)

MODULE 7 REVIEW

1.   D (pp. 533–534)   9.   B (p. 545)

2.   B (p. 534)   10.   A (p. 546)

3.   A (p. 534)   11.   C (p. 557)

4.   B (p. 535)   12.   A (p. 558)

5.   C (p. 537)   13.   C (p. 557)

6.   D (p. 537)   14.   C (pp. 563–565)

7.   A (pp. 541–542)   15.   B (p. 559)

8.   C (p. 542)

APPENDIX 1: DETERMINING YOUR PATIENT'S BLOOD PRESSURE

EXERCISES

1. One of the best ways an EMR can determine the condition of a patient is to identify a trend in the vital signs. A trend can be identified with multiple sets of vital signs taken over a period of time. (p. 570)

2. 128 (p. 570)

3. 140/90 (p. 570)

4. The center of the bladder should be placed over the inside of the upper arm (brachial artery). Be sure the cuff is well above the elbow so that you have access to the brachial pulse point. (pp. 571–572)

5. The diaphragm of the stethoscope should be placed directly over the brachial pulse point. This is found on the medial aspect of the anterior elbow. Use firm pressure when holding the stethoscope in place. (p. 572)

6. **Method 1:** Inflate the cuff to 180 mmHg for males and 120 for children and begin releasing pressure until you hear a sound. **Method 2:** Palpate the radial pulse on the arm with the cuff. Inflate the cuff until you can no longer feel a radial pulse, then increase the pressure approximately 30 mmHg more before releasing the pressure. (pp. 572–573)

7. The systolic pressure is determined by the location of the needle (pressure) at the moment of the first significant sound that you hear. The diastolic pressure is determined by the location of the needle (pressure) for the last significant sound that you hear. (pp. 572–573)

8. Place the cuff as normal. Locate the radial pulse on the same arm as you placed the cuff. Increase the pressure in the cuff until the pulse goes away and then an additional 30 mmHg. Slowly release the pressure in the cuff while watching the gauge. Note the location of the needle when you first feel the radial pulse. This is the systolic pressure. You will not obtain a diastolic pressure using this method. (pp. 573–575)

9. Palpation is used most often when the ambient noise in the environment is so loud that it makes it difficult to auscultate (hear) using a stethoscope. It is also a good technique when you must take a BP on multiple patients quickly. (p. 573)

10. 120/P (p. 575)

REVIEW

1. A (p. 570)

2. B (p. 572)

3. C (p. 573)

4. A (p. 572)

5. C (p. 573)

© 2009 by Pearson Education, Inc. *First Responder,* Eighth Edition, Bergeron et al.

APPENDIX 2: BREATHING AIDS AND OXYGEN THERAPY

EXERCISES

1. (p. 576)
2. (p. 576)
3. A) bag-valve-mask resuscitator; B) pocket mask with oxygen inlet (p. 578)
4. 100 (p. 578)
5. (pp. 586–587)
6. (p. 586)
7. five (pp. 122–125, 586)
8. seal, face (p. 583)
9. (p. 577)
10. 2000; pressure regulator (p. 580)
11. liters; flowmeter (p. 581)
12. (p. 582)
13. (pp. 581–583)
14. (p. 586)
15. (p. 586)

REVIEW

1. C (p. 586)
2. B (pp. 122–125, 586)
3. B (p. 586)
4. A (p. 586)
5. D (p. 586)

APPENDIX 3: PHARMACOLOGY

EXERCISES

1. See Scans A3-1 and A3-2. (pp. 591, 592)
2. A) C; B) A; C) B; D) E; E) D (pp. 593–597)
3. See Scans A3-3, A3-4, A3-5. (pp. 594, 595–596, 598)
4. A) right medication; B) right dosage; C) right patient; D) right route; E) right time (pp. 597, 599)
5. A) oral; B) intramuscular; C) sublingual; D) inhaled; E) endotracheal (p. 599)
6. (p. 589)
7. (pp. 596–599)

REVIEW

1. D (p. 590)
2. C (p. 589)
3. B (p. 590)
4. C (pp. 597, 599)
5. B (p. 599)

APPENDIX 4: AIR MEDICAL OPERATIONS

EXERCISES

1. A fixed wing (airplane) is often more appropriate for longer transports due to the relatively smaller fuel loads that a helicopter carries. (p. 601)

2. A helicopter is an ideal mode for transport requests that are less than 200 miles and when there is a helipad at each end of the transport. (p. 601)

3. A) an accident scene on the highway with multiple injuries; B) a remote area where there is no airport nearby; C) a short transport (hospital to hospital) where there is a helipad at each facility (pp. 600–601)

4. VFR, Visual Flight Rules—these are the rules and regulations that govern flight when the skies are clear and there is no need to fly through clouds. IFR, Instrument Flight Rules—these are the rules and regulations that govern flight during inclement weather when it is highly likely that flight into clouds is necessary. (p. 602)

5. A) close to the patient; B) an appropriate size; C) as flat as possible; D) free of dirt, sand, or loose debris; E) free of overhead wires; F) free of tall trees or poles; G) free of roaming animals (p. 603)

APPENDIX 5: RESPONSE TO TERRORISM AND WEAPONS OF MASS DESTRUCTION

EXERCISES

1. A) (pp. 605–606); B) (p. 606); C) (pp. 607–608)
2. (pp. 608–609)

APPENDIX 6: SWIMMING AND DIVING INCIDENTS

EXERCISES

1. A) airway obstruction; B) cardiac arrest; C) signs of a heart attack; D) head and neck injuries; E) internal injuries; F) hypothermia (p. 611)

2. pull; throw; float; tow (pp. 611–612)

3. neck and spinal injuries if the patient is unresponsive (p. 612)

4. (pp. 612–613)

5. yes (p. 613)

6. jaw-thrust maneuver (p. 614)

7. no (p. 612)

8. head, neck, spine, hands feet, ribs; injuries to any part of the body (p. 616)

9. air embolus (p. 617)

10. (p. 617)

11. (p. 618)

12. (pp. 618–619)

13. (p. 619)

14. personal floatation device (PFD) (p. 610)

REVIEW

1. D (p. 611)

2. B (pp. 611–612)

3. A (p. 613)

4. D (p. 613)

5. C (p. 614)

POSTTEST

1. C (p. 25)

2. B (p. 65)

3. A (p. 120)

4. D (p. 180)

5. A (p. 124)

6. C (p. 215)

7. C (pp. 309–311)

8. B (p. 329)

9. B (p. 29)

10. C (p. 221)

11. C (p. 345)

12. D (p. 282)

13. C (p. 212)

14. C (p. 218)

15. C (p. 46)

16. C (p. 46)

17. A (p. 339)

18. D (p. 346)

19. D (p. 52)

20. A (p. 417)

21. C (pp. 349–350)

22. B (pp. 413–414)

23. C (p. 335)

24. C (p. 343)

25. A (p. 342)

26. A (p. 434)

27. C (p. 207)

28. B (p. 336)

29. A (pp. 351–352)

30. B (p. 547)

31. C (p. 435)

32. D (pp. 339–340)

33. B (p. 436)

34. C (pp. 251, 253)

35. B (p. 85)

36. A (pp. 254–255)

37. D (p. 265)

38. C (p. 437)

39. A (p. 86)

40. A (p. 464)

41. D (p. 452)

42. C (p. 472)

43. A (pp. 467–468)

44. B (p. 462)

45. D (p. 360)

46. C (p. 296)

47. D (p. 278)

48. D (p. 439)

49. D (pp. 290–291)

50. B (pp. 558–560)

Notes

Notes

Notes

Notes

Notes

Notes

Notes

Notes

Notes

Notes

Notes

Notes

Notes

Notes